CURRENT CONCEPTS OF URETHROPLASTY

Edited by **Ivo Donkov**

Current Concepts of Urethroplasty
Edited by Ivo Donkov

Published by InTech
Janeza Trdine 9, 51000 Rijeka, Croatia

Technical Editor Sandra Bakic

Cover Designer InTech Design Team

Additional hard copies can be obtained from orders@intechopen.com

Current Concepts of Urethroplasty,
Edited by Ivo Donkov
p. cm.
ISBN 978-953-307-392-7

For EU product safety concerns:
IN TECH d.o.o., Prolaz Marije Krucifikse Kozulić 3, 51000 Rijeka, Croatia,
info@intechopen.com or visit our website at intechopen.com.

Meet the editor

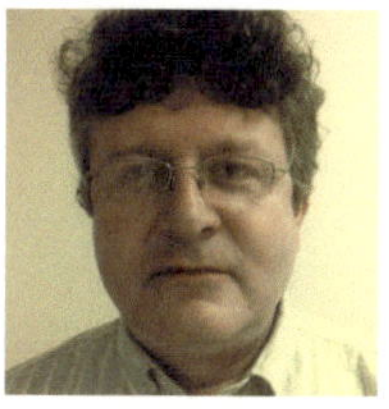

Dr. Donkov is a honorary senior lecturer and honorary academic consultant at the Department of Urology, Medical University of Sofia, Bulgaria. He is also full time urology specialist at Lincoln Hospital, UK. Dr. Ivo Donkov has an abundant profile of specialisations at the most prestigious urology centres of excellence in the world as University College, London, UK and University of California at Irvine, USA. He has passed the American Medical Board, and Canadian Medical Certification exams also. He is on the board of peer review scientific journals and have many publications in peer review journals. Dr. Ivo Donkov is a PhD and his thesis describes biophysiology of different grafts used in urethroplasties, mainly revising the concept of endoscopic urethroplasty, introduced by Jahanes Naude from Cape Town.

Contents

Preface

Urethral reconstructive surgery has always been challenging part for urologist since the dawn of our speciality.

The urethral strictures and defects in development of the urethra (hypospadias and epispadias) are the main issues for urologists, dealing with lower urinary tract reconstructions.

A urethral stricture is a scarred or hardened area that causes narrowing of the caliber of the urethra, and is the commonest problem encountered by adult urology reconstructive surgeons.The stricture eventually reduces or obstructs the flow of urine out of the bladder, making it difficult to urinate. A urethral stricture can occur anywhere in the urethra. Urethroplasty is a surgical procedure conducted to correct scar tissue blockage of the urethra called urethral stricture.

Urethroplasty is a surgical procedure for urethral reconstruction to treat urethral stricture. **Urethroplasty** can be performed by 2 methods; primary repair which involves complete excision of the narrowed part of the urethra, where proximal and distal patent parts are then rejoined. The second method of **Urethroplasty** utilizes tissue transfer of flaps or free graft technique. In this method, tissue is grafted from genital skin, or buccal mucosa and is used to enlarge or replace the strictured (narrowed) segment of the urethra.

The abundance of methods and continuing development of new approaches to the problem prove the complexity of it.

In this book some of the leading experts in lower urinary reconstructions present their views and experience in that field, together with practical tips and tricks. The book is an excellent source of information for those who are already dealing with urethral surgery, and also an invaluable companion for urologists in training or those who want to dedicate themselves to this great sub-specialty.

Ivo Donkov
Department of Urology, Medical University of Sofia, Bulgaria
Lincoln County Hospital, UK

1

Tunica Albuginea Urethroplasty

RK Mathur
Mahatma Gandhi Memorial Medical College & Maharaja Yashwantrao Hospital, Indore India

1. Introduction

The male urethra can be divided into two different portions -The Posterior urethra and the Anterior urethra.The Posterior urethra consist of the membranous and the prostatic part and the Anterior urethra includes the navicularis, penile and bulbous region and is surrounded by corpus spongiosum.

Urethral strictures are an old affliction of mankind and can be defined as "a decrease in the caliber of the urethra due to a scar resulting from tissue injury or inflammation" Usually, fibrosis involves the corpus spongiosum also.

2. Etiological factors

Currently, trauma (accidental or iatrogenic) is the most common cause of urethral stricture. Anterior urethral strictures are caused mostly by the use of indwelling catheters especially the red rubber catheter. Traumatic incidence especially with transurethral resection of prostate has increased the incidence of pendulous and meatal strictures. In developing countries despite increasing awareness and education about sexually transmissible infections (STIs), urinary tract infections also continue to be an important cause and prognostic factor.

Traumatic strictures commonly involve the mucosa and submucosal layers whereas an inflammatory strictures may also extend into the erectile tissue of the corpus spongiosum or the surrounding layers.

3. Techniques available for urethral reconstruction

A wide array of techniques are used in the reconstructive surgery for anterior urethral stricture diseases, and modifications are continuously being made. Stricture excision and anastomotic repair is appropriate only for short and untreated lesions of traumatic origin. End-to-end urethroplasty for bulbar urethral stricture has greater than 95% durable cure rates and low complication rates. Long urethral strictures, which are not amenable to endoscopic correction, require anastomotic urethroplasty.

Urethroplasty of long strictures can be done either by standard two-staged procedures (marsupialization and creation of hypospadias in one stage and closing the lateral skin in midline in a second) or substitution of the strictured part by using genital skin, buccal mucosa and bladder mucosa graft, and so forth. Urethroplasty, with different grafts, usually requires technical expertise and restricture rates are high.

4. Tunica albuginea urethroplasty: A novel technique

Presently buccal mucosal dorsal onlay grafting is considered the standard substitution urethroplasty procedure for anterior urethral strictures. We introduce a technique of anterior urethroplasty by using locally available tunica albuginea of the corpora cavernosa. In tunica albuginea urethroplasty (TAU), the ventral aspect of the tunica albuginea of the corpora cavernosa is used to form the roof of the neourethra.

The anatomical and histological similarity of the tunica albuginea of the corpora cavernosa to the covering of the urethra and its local availability prompted us to use it for urethroplasty. Furthermore, it has been observed that in other cases of urethroplasties with dorsal onlay grafts after necrosis, it is the tunica albuginea that maintains the urethral patency.

5. Tunica albuginea urethroplasty - procedure

5.1 Anatomical remarks

The anterior urethra includes the navicularis, penile and bulbous regions, and is surrounded by the corpus spongiosum. In the bulbar urethra, the relationship between the spongiosum tissue and the mucosal membrane is quite different from the relationship in the penile region: the corpus spongiosum is thick on the ventral urethral surface and thin on the dorsal urethral surface. Furthermore, the urethral lumen is located dorsally and not centrally.

5.2 Operation

The patient is placed in the normal lithotomy position, and a midline penoscrotal incision was given. The bulbar or penile urethra, along with corpus spongiosum, was then freed and was dissected from the corpora cavernosa. The urethra was completely mobilized from the tunica albuginea of corpora cavernosa, which was then rotated and incised along its dorsal surface. The stricture was opened along its whole length.

Thus, the lumen of the strictured segment faced the ventral aspect of the tunica albuginea of corpora cavernosa. An all-silicone urethral catheter was passed through the meatus into the bladder and retained *in situ*. Then, the walls of the slit urethra, along with the tunica of the corpus spongiosum, were stitched to the tunica albuginea of the corpora cavernosa using interrupted vicryl 2-0 sutures at the 5 and7 o'clock positions (Fig. d). Hemostasis was secured and fascia and skin were closed in layers (Fig. e). In this technique, the ventral aspect of tunica albuginea ofcorpora cavernosa forms the roof of neourethra and the floor is formed by a strictured portion of the urethra, along with corpus spongiosum which is cut dorsally.

5.3 Postoperative course

After 21 days, the catheter was removed and a voiding cystourethrography was obtained. Urine culture was repeated every 4 months during the first year and yearly thereafter.

6. Results

Results of the above technique was evaluated in the form of a large scale retrospective and prospective study conducted on 206 patients presenting with symptoms of urethral stricture during the period 1993–2008. After routine workup, in a detailed preoperative assessment, patients were evaluated by means of retrograde urethrogram, urethrosonogram, and uroflometry (preoperatively possible only in cases not having a supra pubic catheter).

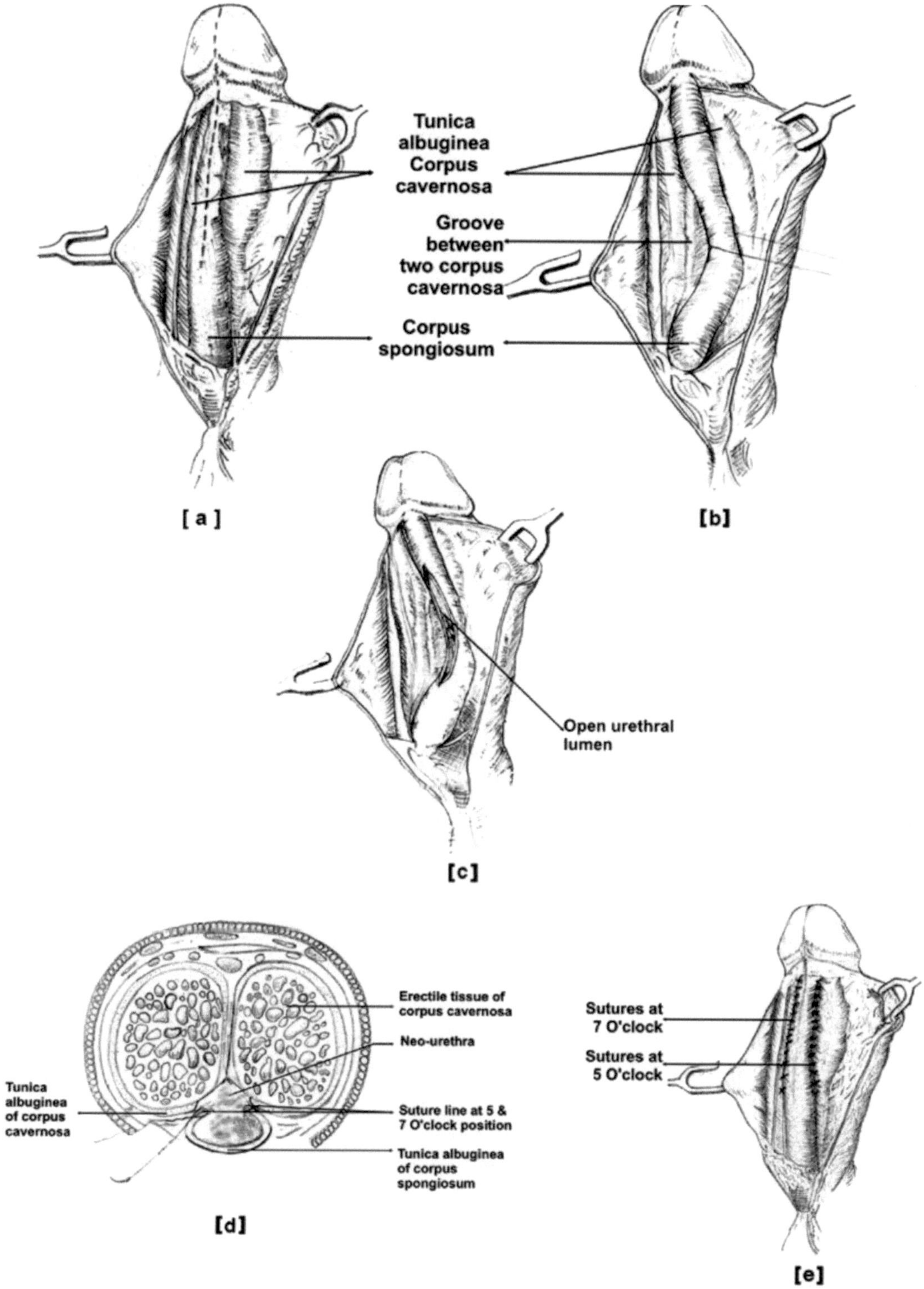

Fig. 1. Technique of Tunica Albuginea Urethroplasty

These patients were taken for TAU, the steps of which are illustrated in the above figure. Among 206 patients, 26 had membranous urethral strictures associated with anterior urethral strictures, which required a combined retrograde urethrogram and micturating cystourethrogram for preoperative evaluation, while in complex cases, magnetic resonance urethrogram was carried out. In all of these patients, U-shaped prostatobulbar anastomosis was carried out along with tunica albuginea urethroplasty.

After surgery, a perurethral 22 French silicon catheter was kept for 3 weeks in simple strictures and for 6 weeks in complex strictures. After catheter removal, patients were scheduled for postoperative assessment with contrast urethrogram, urethrosonogram, and uroflometry. Results were assessed by comparing pre and postoperative investigations and patient satisfaction.

Between July 2007 and September 2008, 30 patients were scheduled for postoperative urethroscopic evaluation. Urethroscopy was carried out only once in these selected patients (in which the outcome had already been assessed by our standard protocol mentioned in. The selection of patients to undergo urethroscopy was random from all groups, so as to allow us to assess both successful and failed cases.

Successful cases were scheduled for urethroscopy to understand how tunica albuginea maintained the urethral lumen without the help of any graft or flap, and also to confirm the growth of urothelium over the area of the roof formed by the tunica of the corpora cavernosa. Failed cases were evaluated to allow an understanding of the process of restricture after surgery.

criteria	**good**	**fair**	**poor**
retrograde urethrogram	Good caliber.	Partial narrowing at stricture site.	Persistent stricture.
urethro-sonogram	Patent and distensible lumen.	Patent lumen with decreased distensibility	Stricture present.
uroflowmetry	Qmax: >20 ml/sec	Qmax: 15-20 ml/sec	Qmax: <15ml/sec
patient's satisfaction	Satisfactory voiding, No instrumentation needed.	Satisfactory voiding but required few dilatations.	Not satisfied, not voiding or voiding with thin stream, need multiple dilatations or repeat surgery.

Table 1. Postoperative result assessment criteria

6.1 Outcome

In the study most of the stricture patients (63%) were young and middle-aged (20–45 years). Among all patients, traumatic and iatrogenic strictures were the most common, followed by infective strictures. Almost 78% of patients had already undergone some previous intervention including multiple urethrotomies, dilations or some form of urethroplasty. Length of stricture (measured intraoperatively) ranged between 2.5 and 12.7 cm with median value 4.6 cm. Mean stricture length was 5.8 cm. It was noticeable that strictures shorter than 2.5 cm were rarely encountered. Probably late presentation for definitive corrective urethroplasty and continued inflammation may be the reason for this. Preoperative uroflowmetry was possible only in 98 patients as more than half of patients had suprapubic catheter for complete urinary retention. Preoperative maximum flow rates (Qmax) analysis showed a range of 3.0 to 12.5 mL/s, mean 7.6 mL/s, mode 5.0 mL/s, median6.8 mL/s and standard deviation of 1.9 cm. Good and fair results were assumed to be successful, while poor results were considered failures. Postoperative and half yearly evaluation showed 96.6% (199) (good85.9% [177] + fair 10.7% [22]) success rate which decreased to 94.7% (195) (good 84.5% [174] + fair 10.2% 21]) at 1 year and 93.2% (192) (good 84% [173] + fair 9.2% [19]) at 2 years. At the end of 3 years, the success rate was over 90% (good 84% [173] + fair 6.8% [14])

Most of the stricture recurrence (14 = 6.8%) occurred within the first 2 years of surgery, followed by 2.4% (five patients) between the 2nd and3rd year of follow-up. A total of 19 cases (9.2%) were considered failures, requiring repeat urethroplasty. Out of the total 19 failed cases, six had lichen sclerosus et atrophicus associated with the stricture and another seven failed cases had combined anterior and posterior urethral strictures. About 10% of patients had minor superficial wound infection, which led to delayed healing. Two patients (<1%) developed urethrocutaneous fistula associated with cases of inflammatory etiology Among 30 patients who were selected for urethroscopy, 18 were good results, seven were fair and five were failed cases.

As visualized on postoperative urethroscopy, in good results, the roof of the neourethra appears to have a similar lining as its base. Hence, it is expected that the urothelium re-grows over the surface of the tunica albuginea. Beyond urethroscopy, the ultimate proof for this can only be a urethroscopic biopsy of the neourethral lining to confirm it is urothelium .In endoscopic evaluation, failed cases showed either circumferential scarring or extensive fibrotic narrowing at the site of reconstruction.

Also supported by studies, preoperative presence of a suprapubic catheter was shown to have a lesser incidence of circumferential scarring at the proximal urethra, as it relieves ballooning of the proximal urethra, drains urine well to relieve urinary stasis, thus ultimately decreasing inflammation in the proximal normal urinary tract.

This probably explains how continued inflammation leaves its mark in the form of fibrosis at expectedly normal ends of the proximal urethra and why there is circumferential scarring as the cause of stricture recurrence after TAU .

Similar fibrotic narrowing was also described by Barbagli *et al.* after bulbar onlay graft urethroplasty in the form of a ring stricture. Failed cases with inflammatory etiology showed diffuse fibrotic narrowing at the site of urethra reconstruction. The entire neourethra lumen was collapsed and replaced by fibrosis as a result of intense inflammation.

7. Advantages of tunica albuginea urethroplasty

Success of free graft apposition depends on neovascularization from the surrounding structures, failure of which leads to necrosis of graft and formation of urethroperineal fistula. Current techniques adopt graft (e.g. buccal mucosa, bladder mucosa) or flap apposition (e.g. pedicled skin flaps, skin island onlay flaps), but this often lacks the mechanical support of a fixed bed, which allows it to fold on itself, reducing the opportunity of neovascularization, and decreasing the caliber of the reconstructed urethra. Moreover, sacculation at the graft side or flap may occur, causing post-voiding dribbling and ejaculatory failure. Sequestration of semen and residual infected urine inside the pseudodiverticulum may further compromise the state of the adjacent urethra and facilitate recurrent stricture disease.

	Good results	Fair results	Poor results
Urethroscopy	Wide patent distensible lumen, regular mucosa	Patent lumen with decreased distensibility, some mucosal irregularities	Distal obliterated lumen, not possible to negotiate scope further

Table 2. Categorization of various urethroscopic findings

Some people recommend that dorsal onlay buccal mucosa graft can overcome these complications, but in a study by Barbagli *et al.* showed that the placement of buccal mucosa grafts into the ventral, dorsal or lateral surface of the bulbar urethra showed the same success rates (83–85%) and the outcome was not affected by the surgical technique.

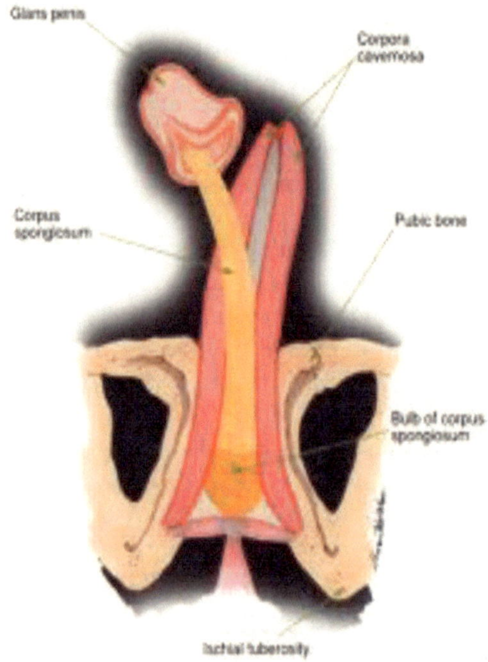

(a)

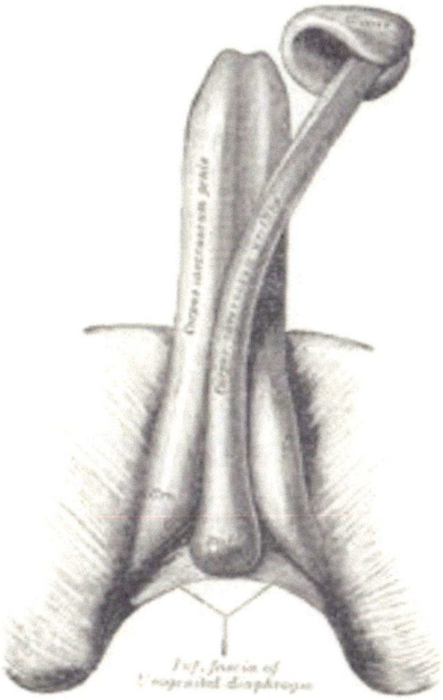

(b)

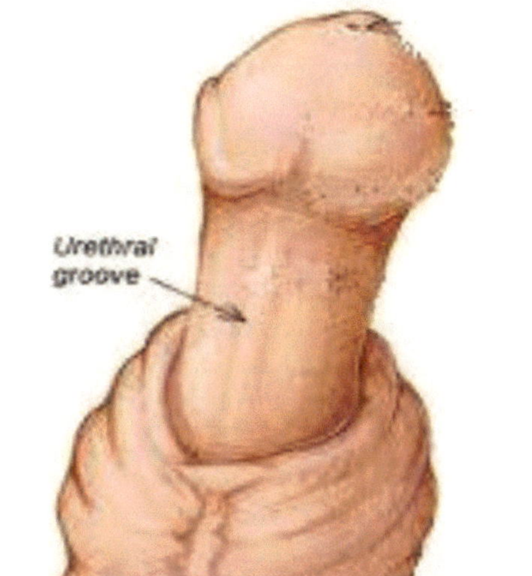

(c)

Fig. 2. Figures showing the urethral groove

The urethroplasty of anterior urethral stricture by using locally available similar structures like tunica albuginea in a single-stage procedure is easy to perform, more feasible and, moreover, anatomically similar tissues are used for approximation as the fibers of the tunica albuginea of the corpora cavernosa and corpus spongiosum are histologically similar in composition and fiber orientation. Both have a circular inner layer that supports and contains the respective cavernous and spongiosal tissues. From these inner layers radiates intercavernosal and spongiosal pillars, respectively, that act as struts to augment the septum, which provides essential support, thus facilitating healing without the dangers of excessive fibrosis which could lead to reformation of the stricture.

The advantages of doing urethroplasty by using tunica albuginea of corpora cavernosa are:

1. Locally available tissue (tunica albuginea of corpora cavernosa) is used.
2. Postoperative restricture rates are very low.
3. The disadvantages of using hair-bearing skin are avoided.
4. It can be used for fairly long strictures (including pan-urethral stricture) without formation of chordae postoperatively.
5. Formation of urethroperineal fistula is not seen.
6. Doesn't require much technical expertise.
7. Cosmetically, the penis looks normal without any bending or curvatures.

8. Conclusion

Urethroplasty, by using anatomically far off and histologically dissimilar grafts, requires more expertise and the chances of restricture are high as well, especially in long strictures. Urethroplasty of anterior urethral stricture by using locally available similar tissue in a singlestage procedure is easy to perform and the postoperative results showed satisfactory results in 94.93% of the patients which is comparable to any other technique. Thus, we strongly recommend the use of tunica albuginea of corpora cavernosa, which is histologically similar and anatomically located near the stricture, rather than using distant and histologically dissimilar tissues such as buccal mucosa, skin and so forth, for anterior urethroplasty.

9. References

[1] Mathur RK, Himanshu A, Sudarshan O. Technique of anterior urethra urethroplasty using tunica albuginea of corpora cavernosa. *Int. J Urol.* 2007 Mar; 14(3):209-13.

[2] Mathur RK, Sharma Adittya K, Sudarshan O. Tunica Albuginea Urethroplasty for anterior urethral strictures. *International journal of Urology* september 2009; 16(9):751-5.

[3] Mathur RK, Himanshu A, Sudarshan O. A technique of anterior urethroplasty using tunica albuginea of the corpora cavernosa. *Asian journal of Surgery* July 2008; 31(3):134-9

[4] Mathur RK, Sharma Adittya K. Tunica Albuginea Urethroplasty for Panurethral strictures. *Urol J.* 2010; 7:120-4.

2

Two-Stage Urethroplasty for Severe Primary Hypospadias

Yun-Man Tang and Shao-Ji Chen
Sichuan Provincial People's Hospital
China

1. Introduction

Surgical repair of hypospadias is challenging and problematic even for the most experienced specialists, and this is especially true when severe and complicated case is confronted. In the history of hypospadiology, surgeons have developed a vast armamentarium of hypospadias repairs that are still in use, with no procedure able to deal with varied cases universally. Debates persist, though the focus of controversies alter. Sometimes we found us involved in a regeneration of old era, an example occasion is that many of us nowadays are faced upon the aroused enthusiasm of two-stage repair for severe hypospadias.

In the early era of hypospadias surgery, two-stage correction with orthoplasty and urethra bed substitution only or as stage I repair, followed by urethroplasty in stage II is a widely accepted strategy in hypospadias repair. The representitive techniques include Denis-Brown procedure and its varied modifications. These techniques are still in use in many centers nowadays (Bar et al, 2005; Brown, 1949; Gearhart & Witherington, 1979; Patel & Caldamone, 2010). The reason of wide acceptance of such techniques is more for technical simplicity tnan for satisfactory function or cosmesis.

In that days, single-stage accomplishment of hyopspadias repair for surgeons was a dream but nightmare concerning the technical poverty and disappointing outcome. It was largely the contribution of John Duckett that the concept and technique of single-stage repair gained worldwide acceptance. The classic transverse prepucial island tube technique became the norm in numerous centers and is still the mainstay for correction of severe hypospadias in many centers currently (Duckett, 2002a, 2002b; MacGillivray et al, 2002; Soutis et al, 2003).

With attention paid to long term outcome and pursuit on cosmesis as time goes on, pitfalls of such island and tube flap urethroplasty in one stage have been seriously concerned by more and more authors. Meatal configuration, glans appearance, limited local tissue for repair, indeed high complication rate in long-term follow-up, the problems such as fistula, glans/neourethra dihiscence, stricture, urethral diverticulum, are all included in criticism and reevaluation. (Castanon et al, 2000; Dermibilek et al, 2001; Dewan et al, 1991; Lam et al, 2005; Powell et al, 2000).

Nowadays, a technique preponderance is obvious in management of mild to moderate hypospadias, ie, application of Snodgrass technique. But for those extremely severe cases, the popular single-stage strategies are still highly problematic. Inspired by free graft techniques used in plastic surgery, some specilists are back to the almost aridit field of two-stage repairs with introducing a free graft as urethra bed for urethroplasty in hypospadias management. The grafts were harvested from extragenital skin, inner prepuce, and evolved to oral mucosa. The latter becomes a new gold standard as urethra substitute in two-stage repair advocated by some authors today (Goyal et al, 2010; Markiewicz et al, 2007; Mokhless et al, 2007; Simonato et al, 2008).

Notwithstanding the dispute on single-stage vs two-stage repairs is ardent, agreement exists that procedure assignment in hypospadias repair is highly based on the patient's individual anomaly status and on the surgeon's individual experience and preference. And, surgical goals are in common, ie, to reconstruct a normal or near-normal appearance mimiking that of a post-circumcision one, to place a water-proof neourethra with adequate and even caliber extending to the apex of the glans for stand voiding and normal urine stream, to create a straight penis adequate for sexual intercorse, and to control the risk of complications (Baskin & Ebbers, 2006).

2. Fundamental requirements in two-stage repair

General process of staged surgery includes adequate orthoplasty, urethra bed preparation and glans/grove augmentation in stage I, and in stage II accomplishment of tubular urethroplasty, meatoplasty, glansplasty, penoplasty and scrotoplasty.

2.1 Stage I

Common requirements in stage I surgery include the follows :

Satisfactory orthoplasty should be achieved in stage I. In most of the severe cases, penile curvature is related to urethral tethering and categorized to group IV chordee (Donnahoo et al, 1998; Mingin & Baskin, 2002; Tang et al, 2007). Plate transection and removal of ventral fibrous tissue is mandatory for orthoplasty in most cases to obtain a straight and length-spared penis, instead of dorsal plication alone.

When plate transection and orthoplasty have been done, usually a large defect between the urethrostomy opening or plate incised margin and subcoronal margin is created. A well urethra bed should be prepared for future tubularization. Neourethral bed is desired to be with appropriate epithelial histological properties withstanding exposure to air until stage II tube urethroplasty, with flat than lumpy surface, with adequate axial length extending to the apex of the glans, with width enough for future retrieval as reconstruction of even and full circumferencial caliber, with good vascularity avoiding acute/chronic ischemia and contracture.

Small glans and shallow groove present in a high proportion of severe hypospadias cases, thus augmentation in stage I is warranted.

2.2 Stage II

In stage II, the aim of surgery is to accomplish the whole correction of the deformities.

In most cases, orthoplasy was satisfactory and the urethal reconstruction becomes the fosus problem. If chordee present as incomplete correction or as recurrence, further management is required.

Urethroplasty is the central problem resolved in stage II correction. With good preparation of urethra bed in stage I, tubularization of the urethra bed for long segment urethroplasty is out of chanllenging. The caliber of the neourethra should be adequate, uniform and similar to the proximal normal urethra. When free graft is the choice of urethra bed substitute in

stage I, graft take should be unquestionable, or else additional tissue should be involved in urethral reconstruction.
To guarantee a water proofing neourethra, an additional vascularized coverage is of great importance.
Relocation of meatus is optimally made on the apex of the glans and be slit-like.
In stage II, a cornical and plump glans is realigned following meatoplasty.
Skin coverage of the penile shaft is required to be smooth in surface, even in axial view, and adequate in length.
Bifid scrotum and penoscrotal transposition are frequently associated with severe hypospadias. Such associated deformities desire correction, usually accomplished in stage II hypospadias surgery. Elemination of scrotal bifida is usually out of problem. While satisfactory correction of severe translocation necessitating radical dissection and may threaten reliability of urethral replacement, thus to leave penoscrotal correction to a future surgery is rational in some cases.

2.3 New concept of two-stage repair

Indeed that the aim of sgate I surgery should be to prepare optimal local anatomic status for stage II other than doctrinal orthoplasty, urethra bed preparation and glans/groove augmentation. Shall we do more in stage I than leave behind so many problems awaiting future resolution? In popular two-stage repair procedures, stage II surgery still bears high risk of complications (Bracka , 2011). This can be explained with the facts that: (1) long segment urethral reconstruction is associated with high risk of fistula, stenosis/stricture, diverticulum/dilatation, and curvature recurrence; and (2) extensive coverage of neourethra as well as correction of bifid scrotum and penoscrotal transposition denotes radical trauma, underlying infection, fascia tethering curvature, and threatened vascularity. Another usual problem of such radical reconstruction, concerning complicated plastic contents vs limited local tissue, is the sacrfice of cosmesis, which has profound psychological disturbance. Some authors tried modifications of the stage I procedure with partial urethroplasty especially in cases owning a relatively long and healthy urethral plate (Schumacher et al, 1997; Cheng et al, 2003). Partial urethroplasty and additional correction of anatomical alterations achieved in stage I surgery might aleviate the reconstructive burden in stage II.
We further advocate a new concept of two-stage hypospadias repair, that two-stage strategy can be either more radical or more conservative (article in press). With technical development and individual experience gathering, one-stage repair of severe hypospadias is advocated by quite a number of specialists, let alone by patients. Our concept of "conservative" denotes that two-stage repair be indicated in those who could be repaired in single-stage, while complicated correction is anticipated with high risk of complications and poor appearance. The concept of "radical" denotes that when two-stage is indicated, much more can be done in stage I to diminish the risks in stage II surgery. In addition to sufficient orthoplasty, partial urethroplasty is achieved distal to the penoscrotal junction, and in some cases extended to the subcoronal area. The defect between neomeatus and the glans tip is substituted with skin flap as urethra bed, meanwhile glans/groove augmentation is accomplished. Stand voiding can be expected with such management. With partial urethroplasty carried out, scrotal bifida is eliminated, penoscrotal transposition resolved in a degree, and penoscrotal angle created. At completion of these steps in stage I surgery, the anomaly becames a much milder variant of hypospadias. Thus reconstruction of stage II surgery is much more easier and much less risky. With twice chances of cosmetic tailor, good appearance can be expected.

2.4 Indications of two-stage repair in severe primary hypospadias

Two-stage repair can be indicated in severe primary hypospadias when: (1) severe chordee (greater than 45 degree) is related to urethral tethering (type IV chodee), and sufficient plate transection warrants long segment urethral substitute; (2) genital skin tissue is insufficient for reconstruction; (3) development of the penis is poor with microphallus and underdeveloped glans/groove, and orthotopic meatus is not likely to be created; (4) severe penoscrotal transposition is associated, with its correction the urethroplasty may be threatened; (5) dorsal hood is not suitable for flap transfer and tubularization in that tissue volume is inadequate, unfolding of prepuce hood endangers vascularity or is dissatisfactory and resulted in a highly irregular surface, or vasculature of dorsal skin is of network type (Yucel et al, 2004); (6) poor cosmesis is expected with single-stage repair; (7) surgeon experience of hypospadias correction is immature (Manzoni & Bracka, 2004; Price et al, 2003; Titley & Bracka,1998). The prevalence of hypospadias is high. The surgical reconstruction is complicated, problematic and this anomaly should be referred to experienced pediatric urologist, pediatric surgeon, general urologist, or plastic surgeon, but indeed a large number of surgeons with less experience are involved in treatment of this disease. Experienced specialists are able to handle varied procedures to deal with individual cases, but for surgeons who manage hypospadias less than 40-60 cases per year, decision-making is difficult. When the less experienced surgeons are confronted with severe hypospadias, a strategy of relatively easy-handled two-stage procedure is a wise choice.

3. Detail concerns in surgery

Practical procedures used in hypospadias varies so greatly that more than 300 procedures are available. To decide which procedure be optimal in individual patient is without consensus, while some common concerns in methodology exist when hypospadias anormaly is disassociated into several deformity parts.

3.1 The nature and severity of chordee

With the aid of intraoperative artifical erection test, the nature and severity of chordee is defined. Chordee, with or without hypospadias, is categorized into 4 groups, namely skin tethering as type I, fibrotic fascia as II, corporal disproportion as III, and urethral tethering as IV (Donnahoo et al, 1998; Mingin & Baskin, 2002; Tang et al, 2007). In most cases of severe hypospadias, the ventral curvature is of type IV or III. Correction of urethral tethering warrants plate transection, chordee resection and urethral substitute. Multiform procedures are used for correction of penile disproportion. Both dorsal and ventral approaches are applicable (Bologna et al, 1999), and currently the most popular procedure is dorsal albuginea plication in the midline area (Bar Yosef et al, 2004; Baskin et al, 2000; Soygur et al, 2004; Yucel et al, 2006). Concerning often poorly developed penis in severe hypospadias, ventral graft is beneficial for shaft lengthening. More radical and complicated procedures including corporeal rotation and penile disassembly are advocated by few authors to correct extreme curvature (Decter, 1999; Mitchell & Bagli, 1996). Additional dorsal plication is nowadays a popular treatment in severe hypospadias with urethral tethering to achieve satisfactory orthoplasty and to save tissue mobilized for urethroplasty.

3.2 Meatus location and morphology

Usually a natural location of the hypospadiac meatus can not represent the severity of the anomaly. This is extremely true in severe hypospadias. When the length of urethral replacement is assessed based on a meatus location, preceding sufficient orthoplasty and urethrotomy on the distal thin urethral are needed. In pinhole meatus, meatotomy is desired.

3.3 Quality of the urethral plate

The urethral plate of severe hypospadias can be fibrotic or relatively healthy. When transected and released, the fibrotic plate contracts dramatically, and removal of the fibrous tissue to the level of healthy urethal is rational. If the plate is healthy and with proper length, it can be preserved as part of urethral substitute. Dense fibrotic band resection also can be resected with elevation of the overlying plate and distal urethra to satisfy orthoplasty and preservation of plate.

3.4 Size and configuration of the glans/groove

A wide groove on flat glans may be preserved intact for stage II urethroplasty, meatoplasty and glansplasty. But in most occasions of severe hypospadias, the glans/groove is underdeveloped with small glans and narrow or shallow groove. Thus glans/groove augmentation is required in stage I. For augmentation, wing dissection of the glans is carried out with either a midline incision or two para-groove incisions. Resurfacing of the raw area with flap or graft leads to effective glans augmentation. When glans/groove size is still inadequate for full circumferential tube urethroplasty in stage II, the strategies of choice may be midline incision as in Snodgrass procedure or, in extreme cases, in stage I to prepare more axial length of urethra bed in the distal shaft area allowing stage II mobilization and advancement, and another wing dissection made to utilize the glans/groove tissue all for meatoplasty and glansplasty.

3.5 Tissue volume, configuration, and vascularity of the dorsal prepuce

As an anatomic feature, preputial skin is defect ventrally and accomodated dorsally to form a hood appearance. The dorsal hood skin is known as the best for urethral reconstruction. Abundant hood tissue may be used to accomplish urethra substitute and penile body skin cover, thus to complete a single-stage repair is possible. But in most severe cases, the tissue obtainable for urethral substiture is limited and a two-stage procedure becomes considerable. Radojicic & Perovic (Radojicic & Perovic, 2004) evaluated the prepuce in hypospadias and categorized the prepuce into 6 groups, namely group A—"monk's hood" or "1 humped" (43 cases, 24.7%), B—"cobra eyes" (80, 45.9%), C—"normal" (intact) (4, 2.3%), D—"flat" (24, 13.8%), E—"v"-shaped (16, 9.2%), and F—"collar-scarf" (7, 4.0%). Cobra eyes and monk's hood prepuces had the most favorable vascular pattern for the creation of flaps, while the "flat" and "v"-shaped prepuces had the most unfavorable vascular pattern. They noted that the flat (group D) and v-shaped (group E) prepuces occur often in severe hypospadias, and the v-shaped prepuce is usually present with penoscrotal transposition. In such cases surgery for hypospadias is even more complicated because the underdeveloped preputium is not appropriate to correct the ventral deficiency. Through a transillumination technique, the prepuce vasculature is recognized and this is of importance in deciding by what manner the prepuce utilized in urethroplasty. Yucel et al (Yucel et al, 2004) classified the arterial vascular anatomy of normal and hypospadiac prepuce as 1 artery predominant, 2 arteries predominant, H-type arching artery and net-like arterial system. They noted that hypospadiac prepuce revealed a net-like arterial system more frequently (50%) and the frequency was higher in more severe hypospadiac prepuce. Such net-like vasculature is not suitable for island tube urethral replacement, and attempt of two-stage repair should be seriously considered.

3.6 Development status of the penis and scrotum

Microphallus is common in severe hypospadias. When this deformity presents, gender assignment, endocrinal mesurement, and the possibility of proper endocrinal treatment should be evaluated prior to surgical correction, especially when bilateral dispalpable cryptorchidism is associated. Only when the gender is assigned as male the correction of hypospadias warranted. Underdeveloped scrotum with bilateral cryptorchidism limits hypospadias reconstruction, then orchidopexy and staged reconstruction of hypospadias are of choice. Preceding endocrinal treatment and orchidopexy are helpful in local tissue augmentation and decrease of complication risk. Sometimes webbed penis can be noted in severe hypospadias. Here the absence of penoscrotal angle appearance is usually resulted from urethral tethering, warranting plate transection. Penoscrotal transpositon is common, and it's presency makes surgical correction of hypospadias more complicated. While scrotal skin with transposition is abundant in many cases, and is useful to supplement the skin coverage of the penile shaft through rotation or advancement flap transfer technique. Properly used flap transfer technique in repair of hypospadias is accompanied with correction of transposition in varied degrees. Dramatical residual transposition after urethroplasty should be left for future correction. Skin in the midline area of bifid scrotum is mostly with mucosa appearance, ie smooth, pinky, and hairless. Such property makes skin in this area a proper candidate to urethal replacement. Apart from midline region utilized in urethral reconstruction, bilateral incision margins should be tailored to eleminate bifida and result in a wound with thick wall to cover the scrotal segment of neourethra and diminish the risk of fistula.

3.7 Neourethral coverage

Neourethral coverage is a guarantee to diminishing risk of fistula. This can be achieved with dartos flap or tunica vaginalis flap (Chatterjee et al, 2004; Snodgrass & Bush, 2011; Tavakkoli Tabassi & Mohammadi, 2010). In free graft two-stage surgery, the dorsal tissue can be set aside for future urethra and skin coverage, then degloving in stage I is unnecessary.

3.8 Skin coverage

To accomplish skin coverage is more of a cosmetic problem than functional one. When this objective is not likely to be succeeded in single stage, staged repairs is desired. To add more tissue in reconstruction for complicated cases, free graft could be involved as well. After stage I correction, the dorsal redundant hood skin is preserved in varied degrees. Thus redundant skin apart from that used in urethroplasty is unfolded and rotated or transposed to cover the penile skin defect. When this is insufficient, usually in the proximal ventral area, mobilization and advancement of scrotal skin may be beneficial.

3.9 Source of free grafts

There is renewed interest in contemporary hypospadiology that the urethra bed be replaced with free grafts. Inner prepuce is the most popular free graft of genitalia origin (Bracka,

1995; Ferro et al, 2002; Johal et al, 2006). In recent years, more and more specilists have recommended utility of extragenital substitute when limited local tissue for repair in severe hypospadias as well as in hypospadias cripple is concerned. The extragenital donors include oral mucosa (buccal, lingual, or labial mucosa), postauricular skin, and skin graft from other donor sites such as abdominal wall and thigh. In general, oral mucosa is the first choice, followed by postauricular skin when oral pathology exists. It is proposed that use of free graft from extragenital origin results in good cosmesis and diminished complication rate (Markiewicz et al, 2007; Mokhless et al, 2007; Tahmeedullah et al, 2003). Some authors propose that all other extra-genital skin graft sites such as groin or inner arm should be avoided altogether. Even when these sites are intrinsically non-hairy, it has been the experience of the authors that skin from these areas when transferred to a highly vascular glans sponge may subsequently start to grow coarse hairs (Bracka, 2008).

4. Surgical techniques of stage I repair

Procedures applied in two-stage hypospadias varies, while two of them are representative and derive multiple modifications. Those two typical procedures are Byars technique and Bracka technique. The procedures vary in stage I, and are similar in stage II with Duplay, Snodgrass, or Snodgraft technique (stage II procedures not illustrated in this chapter).

4.1 Byars technique

Byars technique (Fig. 1) requires orthoplasty through chodee resection and degloving, glans augmentation and urethra bed preparation with Byars flap (bilateral penile skin in continuity with dorsal prepuce) in stage I. The advantage is technical simplicity, and this technique is largely with disadvantage of suboptimal cosmesis.

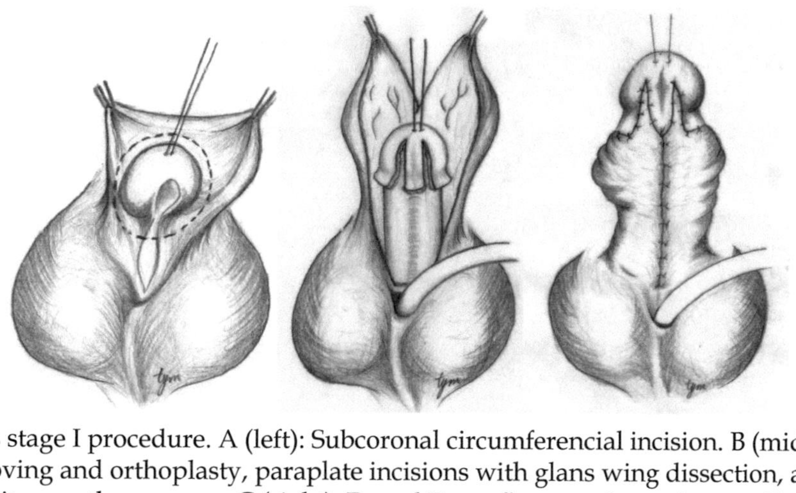

Fig. 1. Byars stage I procedure. A (left): Subcoronal circumferencial incision. B (middle): Penile degloving and orthoplasty, paraplate incisions with glans wing dissection, and dorsal Byars disseciton on the prepuce. C (right): Dorsal Byars flap translocated ventrally to cover the raw area and to prepare urethra bed

4.2 Bracka technique

Bracka previously proposed the use of inner prepuce as free graft for urethra bed substitute, later on he altered his choice to harvest buccal mucosa (Bracka, 2008) (Fig. 2.1 and Fig. 2.2).

With introduction of extragenital graft, room for reconstruction of optimal function and appearance enlarges significantly. The special disadvantages are concerns of donor site mobidities, graft contracture, unsound recipient wound bed, surface keratinization, and absence of long-term evidence for growth synchronism between graft and genital tissue.

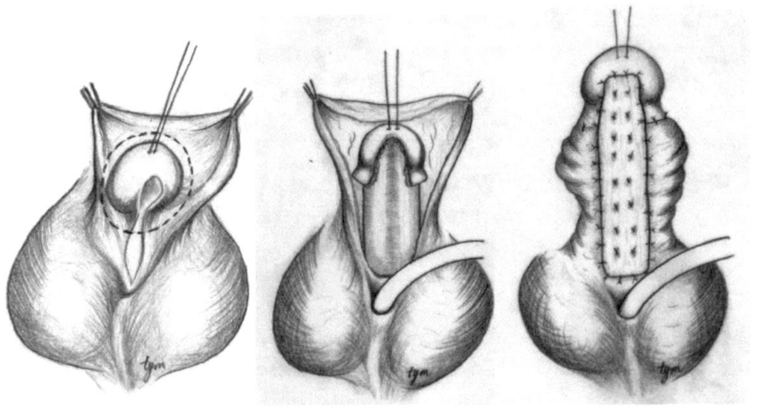

Fig. 2.1 Bracka stage I procedure. A (left): A subcoronal circumferencial incision is made. B (middle): Plate transection, penile degloving and orthoplasty are achieved. With midline incisions on the ventral glans, wing dissection is performed. The axial length and width of urethra bed substitute is measured for preparation of free graft. C (right): The free graft is secured to the ventral aspect of the corpora. Multiple stiches are placed through the graft in order to reduce the risk of hematoma and graft loss

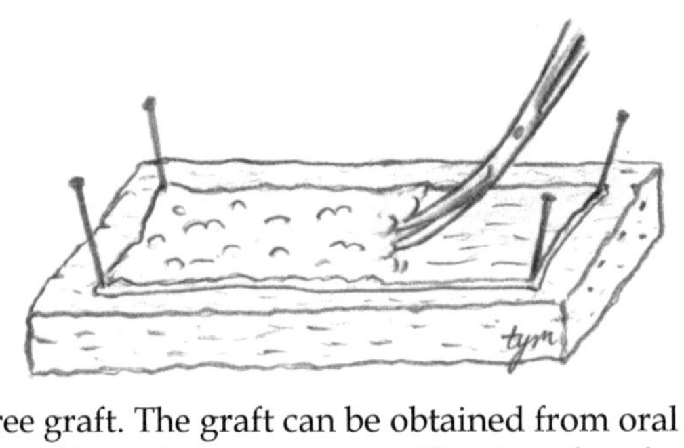

Fig. 2.2 Preparation of free graft. The graft can be obtained from oral mucosa, or other donor sites such as postauricular skin and inner prepuce. The size of graft may be larger than required in case of graft contracture and loss. The harvested graft is placed on a board. Subcutaneous fibrofatty tissue is removed and the graft should be prepared as thin as possible

4.3 Plate reconstruction and tubularization urethroplasty (PRTU) as stage I surgery in two-stage repair

According to the authors' experience, much more can be achieved in stage I. In our team, a two-stage technique in which stage I procedure named as plate reconstruction and tubularization urethroplasty (PRTU) is applied on severe primary hypospadias repair (Chen, et al, 2010; Tang et al, 2010) (Fig. 3.1 to Fig. 3.6). The content of stage I PRTU includes orthoplasty, glans/groove augmentation, partial urethral substitute, urethra bed preparation, correction of scrotal bifida, and correction of penoscrotal transposition in varied degrees

(Fig. 3.1 to Fig. 3.4). Stage II surgery is either a Duplay or Snodgrass procedure. Within a 2 year period, 21 cases with severe hypospadias underwent PRTU surgery as stage I of two-stage repair, and in 14 of them stage II repair accomplished. Followup after stage II repair ranged from 4 to 25 months, with an average of 13.8 months. No fistula, dehiscence, stricture, residual curvature, and dilatation was noted after stage I repair. After stage II repair, distal stricture with urethral dilatation (diverticulum) were noted in 1 case and fistula in 2 (with 1 of the 2 healed spontaneously after 3 weeks saline bath). The patients were otherwise normal in urine stream and cosmesis.

The PRTU technique is versatile in that surgical strategy can be variable with operation proceding. After plate transection and orthoplasty being succeeded, plate reconstruction is performed starting from the meatomy or proximal plate cutting end. Plate reconstruction extends forward and can be stopped anywhere. If the dorsal prepucce is supple and suitable for tube urethroplasty, a combination of island prepucial flap and reconstructed plate tubularization may achieve full circumferencial and full length urethroplasty, ie., single-stage repair is able to be completed. Alternatively, if the dorsal prepuce is moderately deficient, or the configuration and vasculature is not suitable for island tube urethral replacement, reconstruction of plate can be extended to the glans tip and then tubularized, the remaining tissue of Byars flap is utilized for skin cover. Thus a single-stage reconstruction

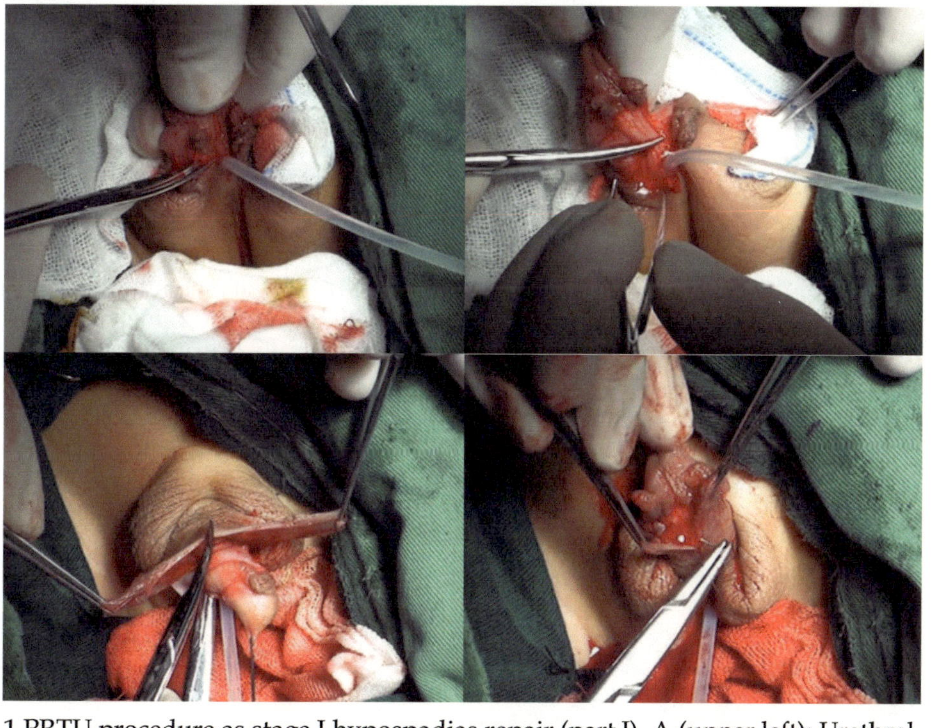

Fig. 3.1 PRTU procedure as stage I hypospadias repair (part I). A (upper left): Urethral transection. B (upper right): Penile degloving and resection of the ventral dense fibrous tissue to correct curvature. C (lower left): Byars dissection on the dorsal prepuce. D (lower right): Byars flaps are translocated to the ventral aspect. Bilateral skin margins were approximated to the midline and sutured together to reconstruct a urethra plate, starting form the meatus/meatotomy opening or transected edge of the natural plate to the penile apex

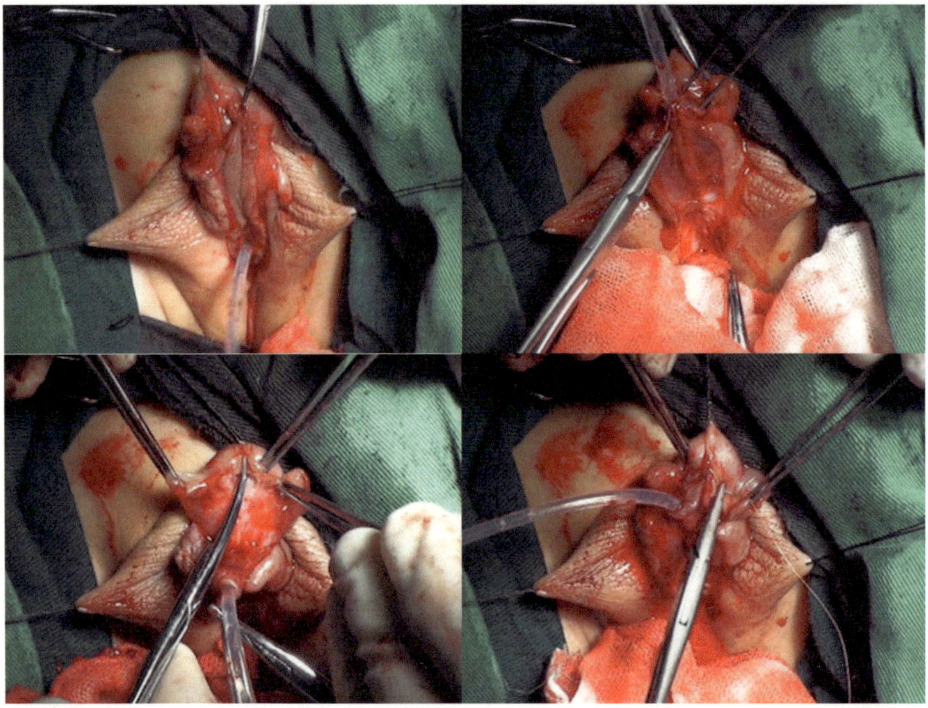

Fig. 3.2 PRTU procedure as stage I hypospadias repair (part II). E (upper left): A U-shaped incision with proper width is made starting form 2 mm proximal to the meatus to the level of anticipated neomeatus, the pecicle vasculature of neoplate is preserved through lateral subcutaneous dissection. The design of neomeatus location is based on evaluation of remaining tissue for skin coverage after urethroplasty (see Fig. 3.3). An alternative strategy to decide the neomeatus location is to extend the incision distally along with tubularization process. F (upper right): Tubularization of the U flap. G (lower left): Midline incision and glans wing dissection. H (lower right): The distal end of ventrally transposed Byars flap is filled in the raw area of wing dissection. The filling flap is trimmed to size for adequate glans/groove augmentation and for future urethroplasty

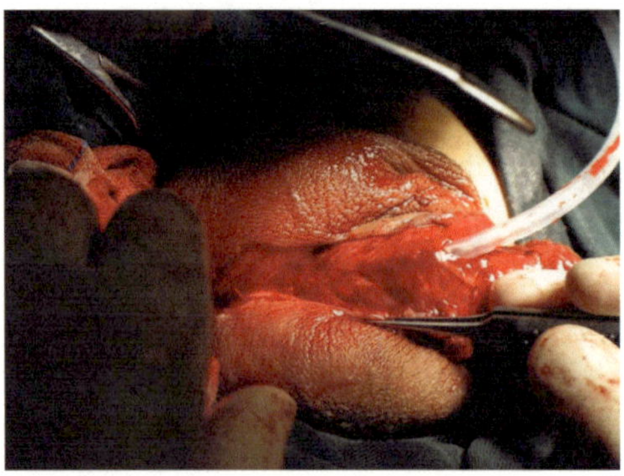

Fig. 3.3 In another case the tube urethroplasty extended to the midshaft and neomeatus created there

is available, too. When the preputial tissue is highly limited and inadequate for both full length urethral replacement and skin coverage, tubularization of the reconstructed plate stops at an appropriate site to allow optimal skin coverage. Thereafter the untubularized part of reconstructed plate as urethra bed is let alone for latter stage urethroplasty.

Advantages of this PRTU procedure include: (1) tissue sparing; (2) good blood supply for neourethra and urethra bed; (3) good cosmesis; (4) well indicated for adult primary repair; (5) relatively simple technique; (6) low complication rate. When genital tissue is extremely limited for reconstruction, disadvantages of this technique may be visualized, ie., PRTU is contraindicated. Introduction of a free graft may be better in this occasion.

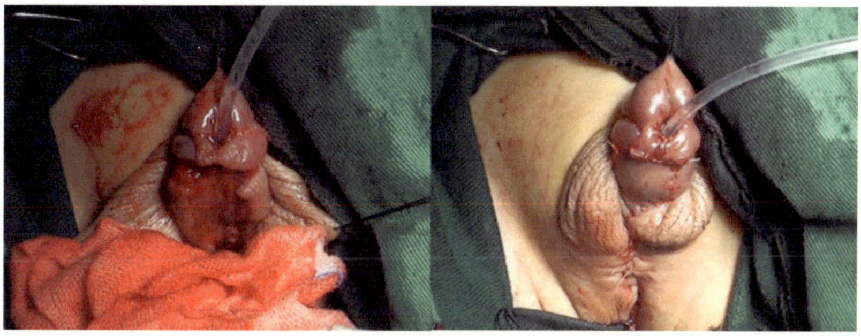

Fig. 3.4 PRTU procedure as stage I hypospadias repair (part III). I (left): The distal end of tube urethroplasty is sutured with adjacent skin to achieve meatoplasty. J (right): Skin cover including penoplasty, scrotoplasty, perineoplasty if needed. Scrotal bifida is eleminated and penoscrotal transposition corrected in a degree

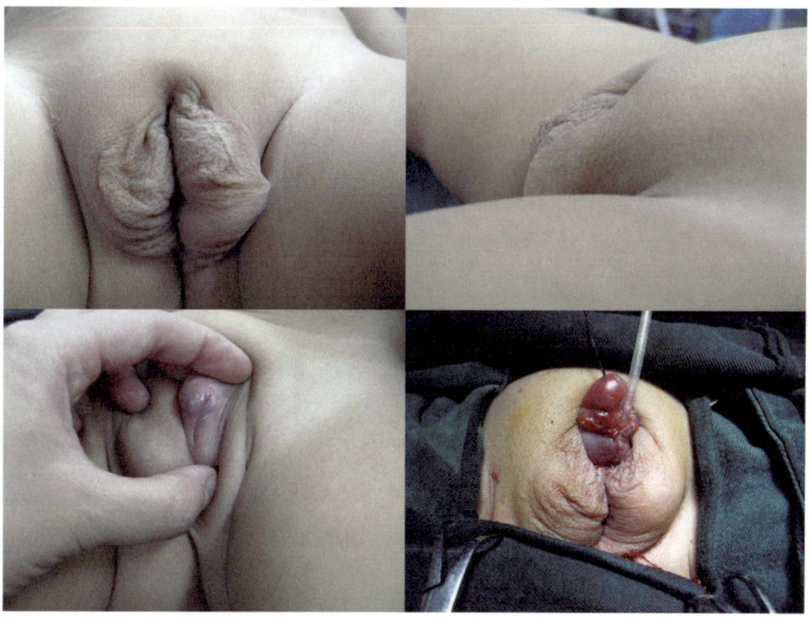

Fig. 3.5 Stage I surgery with PRTU partial urethroplasty in a 2-year-old boy with perineal hypospadias. A. Preoperative front view. B. Preoperative lateral view. C. Preoperative view shows the penis. D. Immediately after stage I surgery

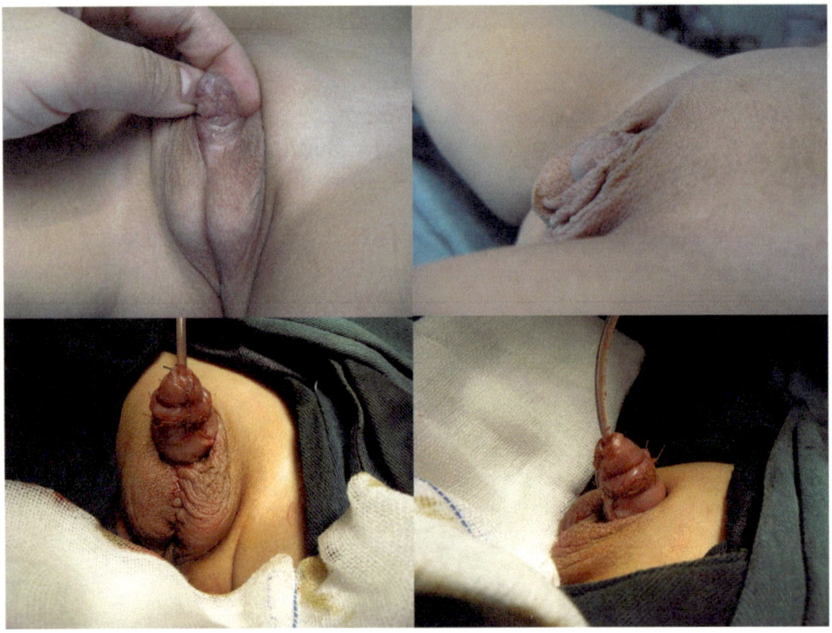

Fig. 3.6 Stage II surgery (with Snodgrass technique) for the same boy 1 year after stage I repair. A. Preoperative front view. B. Preoperative lateral view. C. Front view immediately after surgery. D. Lateral view immediately after surgery

5. The future

In the future, the fact that good cosmesis should be the top goal in hypospadias repair will have great influence on the specialists. Along with technical advance and experience deposition, debate on single-stage or two-stage repair will still exist and hot. As to 2-stage repair itself, progress in regenerative medicine might lead us to a new way, and the concepts such as tissue engineering and stem cells might play some role in our clinical practice (Chen et al, 2000; Atala, 2002; Fossum & Nordenskjöld, 2010; Aboushwareb & Atala, 2008).

6. References

Aboushwareb, T. & Atala, A. (2008). Stem cells in urology. *Nature Cinical Practice Urology*, Vol.5, No.11, (November 2008), pp. 621-631, ISSN 1743-4270

Atala, A. (2002). Experimental and clinical experience with tissue engineering technique for urethral reconstruction. *Urologic Clinics of North America*, Vol.29, No.2, (May 2002), pp.485-492, ISSN 0094-0143

Bar, K., Klijer, R. & Michalak, J. (2005). One-stage urethroplasty for penoscrotal hypospadias using Denis Browne (Michałowski's modification) technique in a 50-year-old man (in Polish). *Wiadomosci Lekarskie,* Vol.58, No.5-6, (2005), pp.335-7.

Bar Yosef, Y., Binyamini, J., Matzkin, H. & Ben-Chaim, J. (2004). Midline dorsal plication technique for penile curvature reapir. *Journal of Urology*, Vol.172, No.4 part 1, (October 2004), pp.1368–1369, ISSN 0022-5347

Baskin, L.S., Erol, A., Li, Y.W. & Liu, W. (2000). Anatomy of the neurovascular bundle: is safe mobilization possible? *Journal of Urology*, Vol.164, No.3 part 2, (September 2000), pp. 977–980, ISSN 0022-5347

Baskin, L.S. & Ebbers, M.B. (2006). Hypospadias: Anatomy, etiology and technique. *Journal of Pediatric Surgery*, Vol.41, No.3, (March 2006), pp. 463-472, ISSN 0022-3468

Bologna, R.A., Noah, T.A., Nasrallah, P.F. & McMahon, D.R. (1999). Chordee: varied opinions and treatments as documented in a survey of the American Academy of Pediatics, Section of Urology. *Urology*, Vol.53, No.3, (March 1999), pp.608-612, ISSN 0090-4295

Bracka, A. (1995). A versatile two-stage hypospadias repair. *British Journal of Plastic Surgery*, Vol.48, No.6, (1995), pp. 345-352, ISSN 0007-1226

Bracka, A. (2008). The role of two-stage repair in modern hypospadiology.*Indian Journal of Urology*, Vol.24, No.2, (April 2008), pp.210-218

Bracka, A. (2011). Buccal mucosa: good but not perfect. *Journal of Urology*, Vol.185, No.3, (March 2011), pp. 777–778, ISSN 0022-5347

Brown, D. (1949). An operation for hypospadias. *Proceedings of the Royal Society of Medicine*, Vol.42, No.7, (July 1949), pp.466-468

Castanon, M., Munoz, E., Carrasco, R., Rodò, J. & Morales L. (2000). Treatment of proximal hypospadias with a tubularized island flap uretroplasty and the onlay technique: A comparative study. *Journal of Pediatric Surgery*, Vol.35, No.10, (October 2000), pp. 1453-1455, ISSN 0022-3468

Chatterjee, U.S., Mandal, M.K., Basu, S., Da,s R. & Majhi T. (2004). Comparative study of dartos fascia and tunica vaginalis pedicle wrap for the tubularized incised plate in primary hypospadias repair. *BJU International*, Vol.94, No.7, (November 2004), pp. 1102-1104, ISSN 1464-4096

Chen, F., Yoo, J.J. & Atala, A. (2000). Experimental and clinical experience using tissue regeneration for urethral reconstruction. *World Journal of Urology*, Vol.18, No.1, (Febrary 2000), pp.67-70, ISSN 0724-4983

Chen, S., Tang, Y. & Mao, Y. (2010). Staged repair for severe hypospadias: Choicelessness? Devolution? Evolution? *3rd World Congress of Pediatric Surgery Abstract Book*, pp. 83, New Delhi, India, October 21-24, 2010

Cheng, E.Y., Kropp, B.P., Pope ,J.C. 4th & Brock, J.W. 3rd. (2003). Proximal division of the urethral plate in staged hypospadias repair. *Journal of Urology*, Vol.170, No.4 part 2, (October 2003), pp. 1580-1583, ISSN 0022-5347

Decter, R.M. (1999). Chordee correction by corporal rotation: the split and roll technique. *Journal of Urology*, Vol.162, No.3 part 2, (September 1999), pp.1152-1154, ISSN 0022-5347

Dermibilek, S., Kanmaz, T., Aydin, G. & Yucesan, S. (2001). Outcome of one-stage techniques for proximal hypospadias repair. *Urology*, Vol.58, No.2, (August 2001), pp.267-270, ISSN 0090-4295

Dewan, P.A., Dineen, M.D., Winkle, D. & Duffy, P.G., Ransley P. (1991). Hypospadias: Duckett pedicle tube urethroplasty. *European Urology*, Vol.20, No.1, (1991), pp.39–42, ISSN 0302-2838

Donnahoo, K.K., Cain, M.P., Pope, J.C., Casale, A.J., Keating, M.A., Adams, M.C. & Rink, R.C. (1998). Etiology, management and surgical complications of congenital chordee without hypospadias. *Journal of Urology*, Vol.160, No.3 part 2, (September 1998), pp.1120-1122, ISSN 0022-5347

Duckett, J.W. Jr. (2002a). Transverse preputial island flap technique for repair of severe hypospadias. 1980. *Journal of Urology*, Vol.167, No.2 part 2, (Febrary 2002), pp.1179-1182, ISSN 0022-5347

Duckett, J.W. (2002b). The island flap technique for hypospadias repair. 1981. *Journal of Urology*, Vol.167, No.5, (May 2002), pp.2148-2152, ISSN 0022-5347

Ferro, F., Zaccara, A., Spagnoli, A., Lucchetti, M.C., Capitanucci, M.L. & Villa, M. (2002). Skin graft for 2-stage treatment of severe hypospadias: back to the future? *Journal of Urology*, Vol.168, No.4 part 2, (October 2002), pp.1730-1733, ISSN 0022-5347

Fossum, M. & Nordenskjöld, A. (2010).Tissue-engineered transplants for the treatment of severe hypospadias. *Hormone Research in Paediatrics*, Vol.73, No.2, (2010), pp.148-52

Gearhart, J.P. & Witherington, R. (1979). The Denis-Browne hypospadias repair revisited. *Journal of Urology*, Vol.122, No.1, (July 1979), pp.66-67, ISSN 0022-5347

Goyal, A., Singh, M.V. & Dickson, A.P. (2010). Oral mucosa graft for repair of hypospadias: outcomes at puberty. *Journal of Urology*, Vol.184, No.6, (December 2010), pp.2504-2508, ISSN 0022-5347

Johal, N.S., Nitkunan, T., O'Malley, K. & Cuckow, P.M. (2006). The two-stage repair for severe primary hypospadias. *European Urology*, Vol.50, No.2, (August 2006), pp.366-371, ISSN 0302-2838

Lam, P.N., Greenfield, S.P. & Williot, P. (2005). 2-stage repair in infancy for severe hypospadias with chordee: long-term results after puberty. *Journal of Urology*, Vol.174, No.4 part 2, (October 2005), pp.1567-1572, ISSN 0022-5347

MacGillivray, D., Shankar, K.R. & Rickwood, A.M. (2002). Management of severe hypospadias using Glassberg's modification of the Duckett repair. *BJU International*, Vol.89, No.1, (January 2002), pp. 101-102, ISSN 1464-4096

Manzoni, G., Bracka, A., Palminteri, E. & Marrocco, G. (2004). Hypospadias surgery: When, what and by whom. *BJU International*, Vol.94, No.8, (November 2004), pp. 1188-1195, ISSN 1464-4096

Markiewicz, M.R., Lukose, M.A., Margarone, J.E. 3rd, Barbagli, G., Miller, K.S. & Chuang SK. (2007). The oral mucosa graft: a systematic review. *Journal of Urology*, Vol.178, No.2, (August 2007), pp.387-394, ISSN 0022-5347

Mingin, G., Baskin, L.S. (2002). Management of chordee in children and young adults. *Urologic Clinics of North America*, Vol.29, No.2, (May 2002), pp.277-284, ISSN 0094-0143

Mitchell, M.E. & Bagli, D.J.(1996). Complete penile disassembly for epispadias repair: the Mitchell technique. *Journal of Urology*, Vol.155, No.1, (January 1996), pp.300-304, ISSN 0022-5347

Mokhless, I.A., Kader, M.A., Fahmy, N. & Youssef, M. (2007). The multistage use of buccal mucosa grafts for complex hypospadias: histological changes. *Journal of Urology*, Vol.177, No.4, (April 2007), pp.1496-1499, ISSN 0022-5347

Patel, S.R. & Caldamone, A.A. (2010). Sir Denis Browne: contributions to pediatric urology. *Journal of Pediatric Urology*, Vol.6, No.5, (October 2010), pp.496-500

Powell, C.R., McAleer, I., Alagiri, M. & Kaplan GW. (2000). Comparison of flap versus grafts in proximal hypospadias surgery. *Journal of Urology*, Vol.163, No.4, (April 2000), pp.1286-1288, ISSN 0022-5347

Price, R.D., Lambe, G.F. & Jones, R.P. (2003). Two-stage hypospadias repair: Audit in a district general hospital. *British Journal of Plastic Surgery*, Vol.56, No.8, (December 2003), pp. 752-758, ISSN 0007-1226

Radojicic, Z.I. & Perovic, S.V. (2004). Classification of prepuce in hypospadias according to morphological abnormalities and their impact on hypospadias repair. *Journal of Urology*, Vol.172, No.1, (July 2004), pp.301-304, ISSN 0022-5347

Schumacher, S., Yabumoto, H., Salge, S., Shrestha, G. & Ikoma F. (1997). Surgical results of complete hypospadias repair in two stages. *International Urology and Nephrology*, Vol.29, No.3, (1997), pp.333-40

Simonato, A., Gregori, A., Ambruosi. C., Venzano, F., Varca, V., Romagnoli, A. & Carmignani, G. (2008). Lingual mucosal graft urethroplasty for anterior urethral reconstruction. *European Urology*, Vol.54, No.1, (July 2008), pp.79-85, ISSN 0302-2838

Snodgrass, W. & Bush, N. (2011). Tubularized incised plate proximal hypospadias repair: Continued evolution and extended applications. *Journal of Pediatric Urology*, Vol.7, No.1, (Febrary 2011), pp.2-9

Soutis, M., Papandreou, E., Mavridis, G. & Keramidas, D. (2003). Multiple failed urethroplasties: definitive repair with the Duckett island-flap technique. *Journal of Pediatric Surgery*, Vol.38, No.11, (November 2003), pp. 1163-1166, ISSN 0022-3468

Soygur, T., Filiz, E., Zumrutbas, A.E. & Arikan, N. (2004). Results of dorsal midline plication in children with penile curvature and hypospadias. *Urology*, Vol.64, No.4, (October 2004), pp.795-798, ISSN 0090-4295

Tahmeedullah, Khan, A. & Obaidullah MA. (2003). Comparison of preputial skin, postauricular skin and buccal mucosal graft results in hypospadias repair. *Journal of the College of Physicians and Surgeons – Pakistan*, Vol.13, No.9, (September 2003), pp.515-518

Tang, Y.M., Chen, S.J., Huang, L.G. & Wang, M.H. (2007). Chordee without hypospadias: report of 79 Chinese prepubertal patients. *Journal of Andrology*, Vol.28, No.4, (July-August 2007), pp.630-633, ISSN 0196-3635

Tang, Y., Chen, S., Mao, Y., et al. (2010). Plate reconstruction and tubularization for correction of severe hypospadias, *3rd World Congress of Pediatric Surgery Abstract Book*, pp. 84, New Delhi, India, October 21-24, 2010

Tavakkoli Tabassi, K. & Mohammadi, S. (2010). Tunica vaginalis flap as a second layer for tubularized incised plate urethroplasty.*Urology Journal*, Vol.7, No.4, (Fall 2010), pp.254-257

Titley, O.G. & Bracka, A. (1998). A 5-year audit of trainees experience and outcomes with two-stage hypospadias surgery. *British Journal of Plastic Surgery*, Vol.51, No.5, (July 1998), pp.370-375, ISSN 0007-1226

Yucel, S., Guntekin, E., Kukul, E., Karaguzel, G., Ciftcioglu, A., Melikoglu, M. & Baykara, M. (2004). Comparison of hypospadiac and normal preputial vascular anatomy.

Journal of Urology, Vol.172, No.5 part 1, (November 2004), pp.1973-1976, ISSN 0022-5347

Yucel, S., Sanli, A., Kukul, E., Karaguzel, G., Melikoglu, M. & Guntekin, E. (2006). Midline dorsal plication to repair recurrent chordee at reoperation for hypospadias surgery complication. *Journal of Urology*, Vol.175, No.2, (Febrary 2006), pp.699-702, ISSN 0022-5347

3

Versatility of Tubularized Incised Plate Urethroplasty in Management of Different Types of Hypspadias

Gamal Al-Saied
Al-Azhar University, Cairo,
Egypt and King Abdul Aziz Specialist Hospital, Taif
Saudi Arabia

1. Introduction

Hypospadias is one of the most common congenital anomalies occurring in approximately 1 of 200 to 1 of 300 live births.(1) Many operations have been described for repair of hypospadias. The introduction of Tubularized Incised-Plate (TIP) urethroplasty by Snodgrass in 1994 have resulted in a revolution in management of different types of hypospadias (distal and proximal either new cases or re-operative cases) as documented by many reports.(2-7) The purpose of this review article is to emphasize that TIP urethroplasty with neourethral coverage using a vascularized pedicled flap of dartos fascia is versatile and simple operation with good functional and cosmetic outcome.

2. Surgical technique

Under complete a septic technique, a traction suture of 5-0 silk is placed in the glans to stabilize the penis during the procedure and help in demonstration of the abnormal curvature and redundant dorsal preputial skin. A circumscribing incision is made 2 mm proximal to the hypospadiac meatus, and the penis is degloved to the penoscrotal junction in cases with proximal meatus. In cases of hypoplastic urethra (the urethra devoid of corpus spongiosum), the meatus is preserved in all patients by a de-epithelialization of hypoplastic urethra. Artificial erection is conducted to verify the penile shaft without bending. If the penis is straight, TIP repair is continued; parallel longitudinal incisions are then made approximately 6 to 8 mm apart to separate the glans from the lateral margins of the plate and the glanular wings are mobilized to facilitate subsequent glans closure without tension. Then, the edges of the urethral plate are gently retracted laterally with fine forceps to delineate the midline which is deeply incised with tenotomy scissors from the hypospadiac meatus to the end of the plate, just below the tip of glans penis [Figure 1]. The incised urethral plate is tubularized without tension over a catheter of an appropriate size [6Fr or 8Fr], using two-layer 6/0 polyglactin sutures, (first layer is running sub-epithelial and second layer is interrupted sub-epithelial suture), [Figure 2]. The epithelium of the urethral plate is

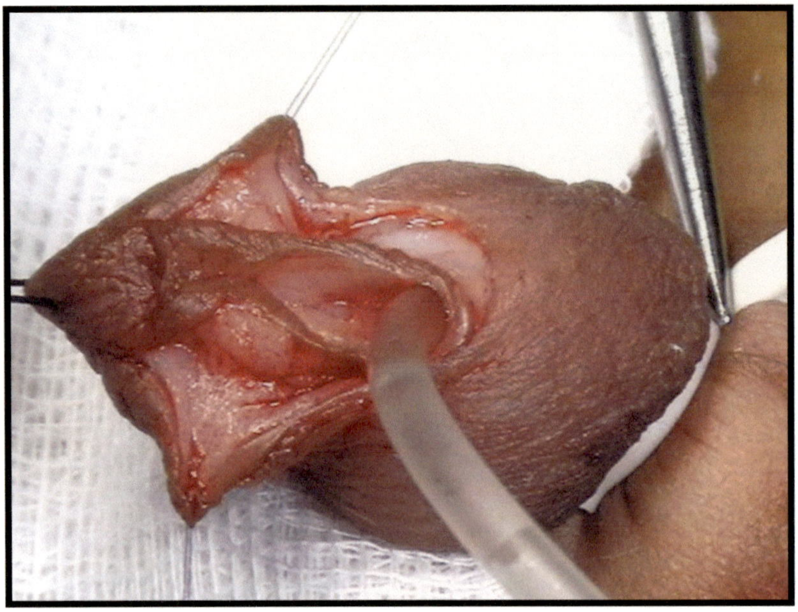

Fig. 1. A U-shaped skin incision is made surrounding the meatus and paramedian incisions are made bilaterally along the urethral plate. The urethral plate is incised sufficiently deeply in its midline from just below the tip of the glans to the regressed meatus

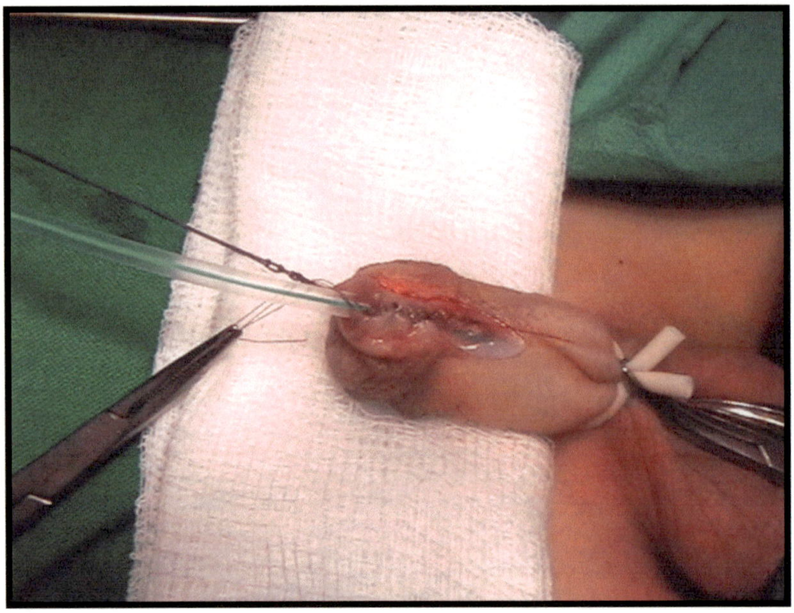

Fig. 2. The incised urethral plate (TIP) is tubularized without tension over a catheter of an appropriate size ,using two-layer 6/0 polyglactin sutures (1st layer is running sub-epithelial and 2nd layer is interrupted sub-epithelial suture). Then the corpus spongiosum alongside the plate is sutured together over the neourethra with the "Y to I" technique

inverted toward the lumen to avoid fistula formation. Then, the corpus spongiosum alongside the plate is sutured together over the neourethra with the "Y to I" technique. In all cases, a vascularized dartos fascia flap harvested either from the prepuce or the penile shaft was used to cover the urethroplasty as a second layer. It is placed in such a manner as to cover the original suture line and sutured with periurethral tissue. Care must be taken to avoid rotation of the penis [Figure 3]. Then, the lateral glans wings are re-approximated over the neourethra using vertical mattress 6/0 polyglactin sutures [Figure 4].

If the curvature is less than 30 degree, dorsal plication of the corporal tissue in the midline is performed to preserve the urethral plate [Figure 5 and 6]. In case of severe chordee more than 30 degree, excision of the chordee followed by covering of the ventral raw area with preputial or penile shaft skin as a first stage. Then, after 6 months, the neo-urethra is fashioned from the healthy skin over a catheter of an appropriate size starting from the hypospadiac meatus and continued distally with incised urethral plate of the glans.

Then, Preputial skin is divided in midline and rotated on both sides of the shaft of the penis to cover the second layer of dartos fascia and sutured to the subglandular skin edge to cover the ventrum of the penis. In circumcised patients, penile ventral skin is approximated and sutured to cover the ventrum of the penis. Then, a straight catheter within the urethra was secured distally to the glans with the traction suture. The duration of the catheter indwelling ranges from 7 to 10 days according to the length of the neourethral. A compression dressing is applied and the first change of dressing is performed 48 hours after surgery to assess the viability of the repair and to detect the acute postoperative complications (bleeding, haematoma and oedema). Prophylactic IV antibiotic (3rd generation cephalosporin) started 30 minutes before induction of anesthesia and continued for 48 hours postoperatively. All patients were kept on regular follow up in outpatient clinic at the end of first, third and sixth month postoperatively.

3. Discussion

A technique to repair hypospadias with universal applicability in most variants would be appealing. The Snodgrass technique is a simple technical innovation that has revolutionized hypospadias surgery. Rich et al.,(1989) first described an incision in the urethral plate to obtain a cosmetically acceptable vertical slit-like meatus for the Mathieu repair.(8) This was subsequently adopted for the entire length of the urethral plate as a complement to the Thiersch-Duplay urethroplasty for distal hypospadias reported by Snodgrass.(2-5) The dorsal relaxing incision over the urethral plate results in a neourethra of more than 10 F (2-5) and does not seem to compromise the blood supply of urethral plate.(9-10) It also results in re-epithelialization rather than fibrosis of the subcutaneous tissue which may later give rise to stricture of the neourethra.(4,6,11) In 2001, Borer et al., found that the risk of fistula was reduced by using second layer to cover the suture line, and recommend this maneuver after TIP urethroplasty.(6) In 2003, Samuel and Wilcox used a second layer of vascularized pedicle subcutaneous tissue harvested from the dorsal hooded prepuce provided cover for the urethroplasty to minimize the incidence of urethrocutaneous fistula.(7) In 2003, Sozubir and Snodgrass mentioned that dartos pedicle flap obtained from the dorsal prepuce and shaft skin is used to cover the neourethra. In some patients with proximal hypospadias, the corpus spongiosum alongside the plate is sutured together over the neourethra with the "Y to I" technique before the dartos flap is applied.(12-13)

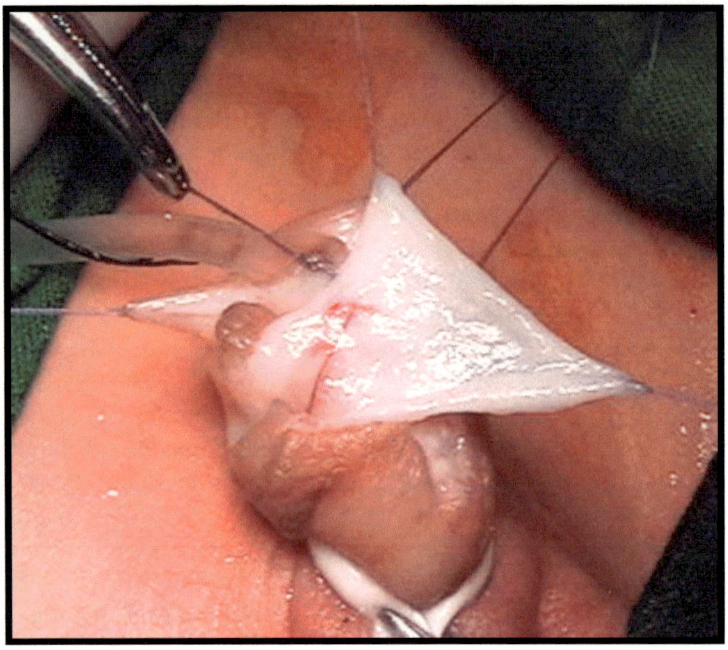

Fig. 3. A vascularized dartos fascia flap harvested from the prepuce is used to cover the neourethra as a second layer

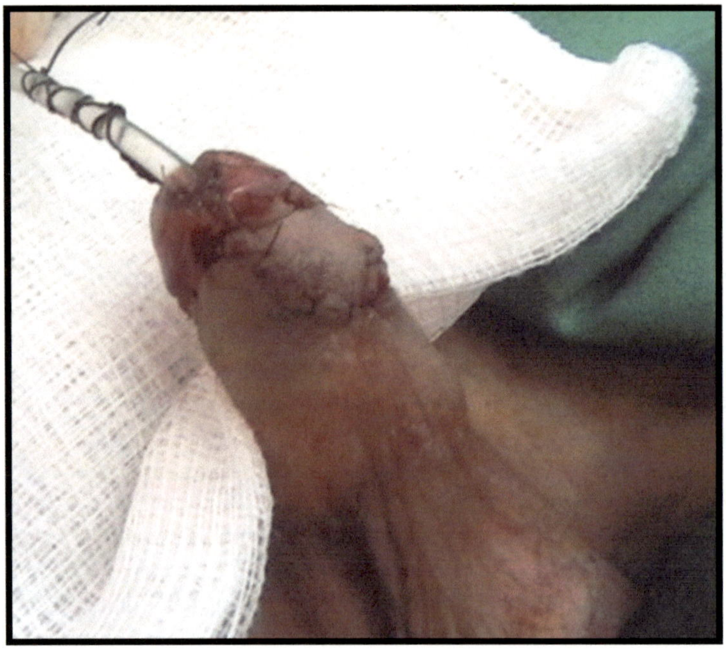

Fig. 4. After the lateral glans wings are reapproximated over the neourethra, the ventral aspect of the penis is covered with penile prepuce, which is sutured to the subglanular skin edge

In 2002, Elbakry concluded that post operative regular urethral calibration should be considered as an integral part of the TIP urethroplasty to prevent the neourethral and/or meatal stenosis with subsequent urethral fistula.(14)
In 2002 Lorenzo and Snodgrass concluded that dilatation of the neourethra is unnecessary after TIP urethroplasty and the calibration and uroflowmetry 6 months after surgery may be useful to detect subclinical obstruction. They attributed the meatal stenosis detected in other series (Elbakry 2002) to the technical error including failure to deeply incise the plate and/or tubularization of urethral plate too far distally.(15)
In our series, the urethrocutaneous fistula was seen in 6(4.14%) of 1ry(new) cases and 5(16.67%) of 2ry (previously failed repair) cases. Meatal stenosis, urethral stricture and meatal regression were observed in 17(9.71%), 5 (2.86%), and 10 (5.71%) respectively, inspite of the deep incision of urethral plate and tension free tubularization of urethral plate to a adequate length. All cases of urethral stricture and most cases of meatal stenosis responded well to regular urethral dilatation. Meatoplasty was performed in only 5 (2.85%) cases (1 of 1ry cases and 4 of 2ry cases). Secondary surgery for fistula repair was successful in all patients (19)
In 2002 Snodgrass and Lorenzo concluded that TIP urethroplasty can be used for hypospadias reoperation, even when the urethral plate has been incised previously, but should be avoided when the urethral plate is obviously scarred or has been resected.(16)
TIP urethroplasty was used for hypospadias reoperation with successful results.(19)
Thin distal urethra devoid of spongiosum sometimes called 'hypoplastic urethra has been noticed in approximately one-fourth of patients undergoing urethroplasty.(17) In our series, the hypoplastic urethra was observed in 25(17.24%) cases.(19)
Traditionally, the hypoplastic urethra is spatulated till the 'healthy' urethra with spongiosum cover is obtained and the urethroplasty is commenced. This step creates a more proximal hypospadias, thus increasing the chances of postoperative fistula.(18)
In our series, the urethral hypoplasia is preserved by its de-epithelialization. De-epithelialization starts venterally and proximally at the normal penile skin below the hypospadiac meatus. At this site,dissection of subcutaneous tissue is facilitated by injection of few ml of normal saline using a fine needle (insulin needle) to achieve separation of adherent skin from the urethra and continues distally up to hypospadiac meatus. Then, the neourethra is reinforced by suturing the corpus spongiosum alongside the plate together over the neourethra with the "Y to I" technique before the dartos flap is applied with good functional and cosmetic outcome.(19)
In case of severe chordee more than 30 degree of 1ry cases, or scarred urethral plate of 2ry cases, the chordee or fibrosed urethral plate is excised and the ventral raw area is covered with either preputial or penile shaft skin as a first stage. Then, after 6 months, the neo-urethra is fashioned from the healthy skin over a catheter of an appropriate size, starting from the hypospadiac meatus and continued distally with incised urethral plate of the glans.(19)
In conclusion, the good functional and cosmetic outcome of TIP urethroplasty are attributed to; 1) tension free fashioning of the neo-urethra from the healthy urethral plate (non-scarred) over a catheter of an appropriate size, 2) using of two layers of 6/0 polyglactin sutures, (first layer is running sub-epithelial and second layer is interrupted sub-epithelial suture), with aid of magnification tools, 3) suturing of the corpus spongiosum alongside the plate together

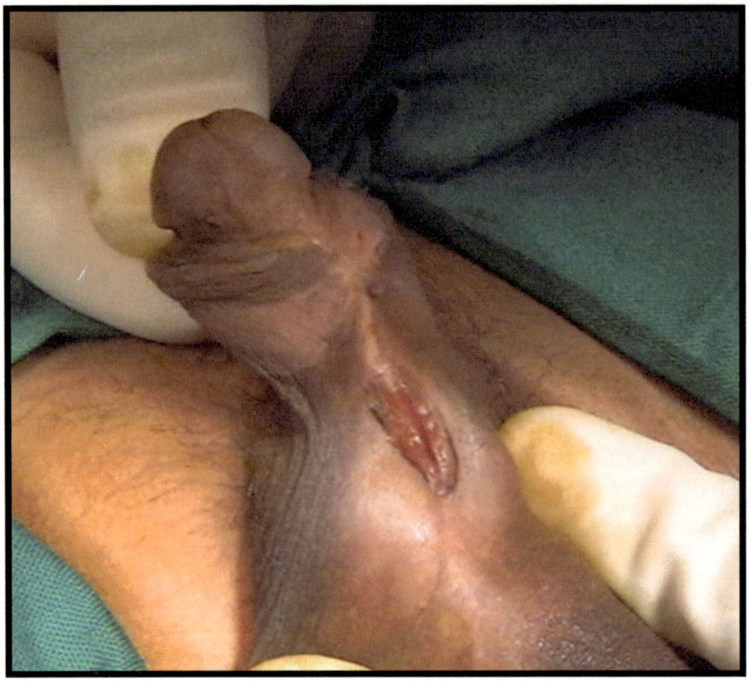

Fig. 5. Penoscrotal hypospadias with chordee less than 30 degree

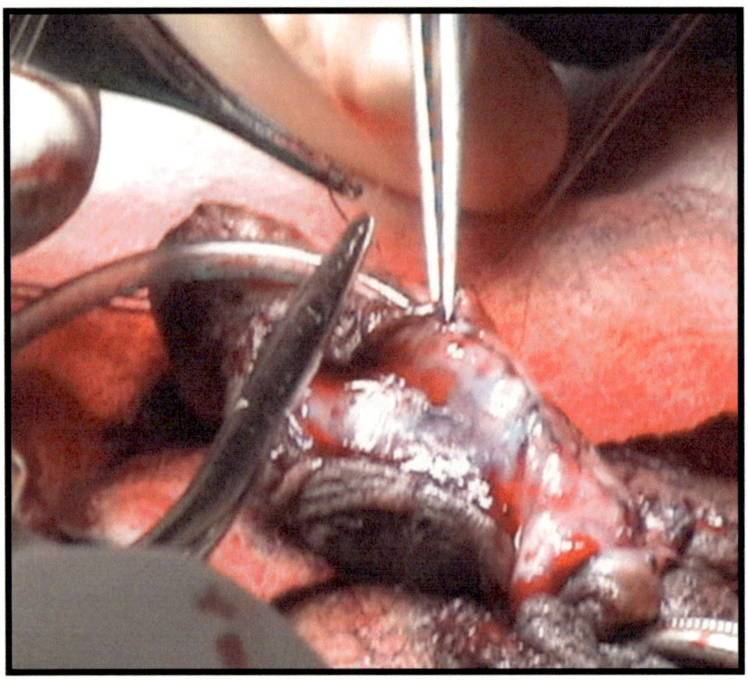

Fig. 6. Dorsal plication of the corporal tissue is done in the midline to preserve the urethral plate then, TIP urethrolplasty is performed

over the neourethra with the "Y to I" technique, 4) and application of second layer of vascularized dartos pedicle flap harvested either from the dorsal prepuce or penile shaft skin in circumcised patients to cover the suture line after TIP urethroplasty.

4. References

[1] Baskin LS, Colborn T, Himes K. Hypospadias and endocrine disruption: is there a connection? *Environ Health Perspect* 2001;109:1175-83.

[2] Snodgrass W. Tubularized incised plate urethroplasty for distal hypospadias. JL/ro/1994; 151:464-5

[3] Snodgrass W, Koyle M, Manzoni G,Horowitz R, Caldamone A, Ehrlich R. Tubularized Incised Plate hypospadias repair, results of a multicenter experience. *J Uro/*1996; 156:839-41

[4] Snodgrass W, Koyle M, Manzoni G,Horowitz R, Caldamone A, Ehrlich R. Tubularized Incised Plate hypospadias repair for proximal hypospadias. *J Uro/*1998; 159:2129-31

[5] Snodgrass W. Does Tubularized Incised Plate hypospadias repair create neourethra strictures?. *J Urol* 1999; 162:1159-61

[6] Borer JG, Bauer SB, Peters CA, DiamondDA, Atala A, Cilento BG. Tubularized incised plate urethroplasty. Expanded use in proximal and repeat surgery for hypospadias. *J Urol* 2001; 165: 581 -5

[7] Samuel M. and Wilcox DT. Tubularized incised-plate urethroplasty for distal and proximal hypospadias *BJU Int* 2003; 92: 783-785

[8] Rich MA, Keating MA, Snyder HM III, Duckett JW. Hinging the urethral plate in hypospadias meatoplasty. *J Urol* 1989; 142:1551-3

[9] Baskin LS, Erol A, Ying WL, Cunha GR.Anatomic studies of hypospadias. *J Uroi* 1998; 160: 1108-15

[10] Erol A, Baskin LS, Li YW, Liu WH. Anatomical studies of the urethral plate: why preservation of the urethral plate is important in hypospadias repair. *BJU Int* 2000; 85: 728-34

[11] Horasanii K, Perk C, Yesildere T. The effect of catheterization time on tissue regeneration after a deep urethral plate incision. *BJU int 2000;* 87:20

[12] Sozubir S. and Snodgrass W.: A new algorithm for primary hypospadias repair based on tip urethroplasty. *J Pediatric Surg* 2003; 38:1157-1161

[13] Yerkes EB, Adams MC, Miller DA, et al. Y-to-I wrap: Use of the distal spongiosum for hypospadias repair. *J Urol* 2000; 163:1536.

[14] Elbakry A: further experience with Tubularized-incised urethral plate technique for hypospadias repair, 2002; *BJU Int* 89:291-294

[15] Lorenzo A and Snodgrass W. Regular dilatation is unnecessary after Tubularized incised plate hypospadias repair. *BJU Int.* 2002; 89:94-97

[16] Snodgrass W.T. and Lorenzo A.J. Tubularized incised-plate urethroplasty for hypospadias reoperation. 2002; *Br J Urol Int* 89:98-100.

[17] Yang SS, Chen YT, Hsieh CH, Chen SC. Preservation of the thin distal urethra in hypospadias repair. *J Urol* 2000; 164:151-3.

[18] Sarin YK, Manchanda V. Preservation of urethra devoid of corpus spongiosum in patients undergoing urethroplasty. *Indian J Urol* 2006; 22:326-8

[19] Al-Saied G and Gamal A. Versatility of tubularized incised plate urethroplasty in the management of different types of hypospadias: 5-year experience. *Afr J Paediatr Surg* 2009; 6:88-92

4

Urethroplasty; Wide Range of Therapeutic Indications and Surgical Techniques

Mahmoud Mustafa[1], Dina Abugaber[2], Sacit Nurigorgel[3], Ertugrul Sefik[3], Ozan Horsanali[3] and Wael Sadaqah[2]
[1]An-Najah University, School of Medicine, Urology Department, Nablus-West-Bank,
[2]Rafidia State Hospital, Intensive Care Unit, Nablus-West-Bank,
[3]Izmir Ataturk Teaching Hospital, Urology Department, Izmir
[1,2]Palestine
[3]Turkey

1. Introduction

Urethroplasty means plastic surgery of the urethra. Herein we are going to describe urethroplasty in terms of; diagnosis, indications, surgical techniques and definition of failure or success. A lot of issues related to urethroplasty remain to be defined, therefore we will clarify the debatable issues and highlight the last advances on urethroplasty.

There are two main causes which mandate urethroplasty; the first is the congenital anomalies with hypospadias being the most common, and the acquired anomalies with urethral stricture being the most common of them. Hypospadias is found commonly in newborn boys and it seen in approximately 8.2 per 1000 births. The goal of hypospadias reconstruction are to bring the meatus close to glans to allow the child to void standing, removing the chordee to allow for normal sexual intercourse and giving the phallus appearance of a normally circumcised penis when observed from distance. There are more than 200 named surgical procedure to correct hypospadias. Now a days tubularized incised plate (TIP) urethroplasty described by Snodgrass in 1994 is the most common procedure used for repair of hypospadias. The advantages of this technique include its simplicity, high success rate, low rate of complication and excellent cosmetic results. A lot of modifications were introduced on the TIP urethroplasty aiming to improve the success rate and to decrease fistula formation. We were from the firsts who published such modification regarding the use of double- layer dartos flap covering for urethra instead of the classic way of utilizing dorsal dartos flap (button hole maneuver).

The second cause of urethroplasty is the acquired anomalies. Strictures of urethra is of much clinical important than hypospadias, because it bothers the patients more, unfortunately the results of surgery is not promising as that of hypospadias. The term “urethral stricture” refer to anterior urethral disease or scaring process involving the spongy erectile tissue of the corpus spongiosum (spongiofibrosis). According to World Health Organization posterior urethral stricture are not included in the common definition of urethral stricture and the term stricture is limited to the anterior urethra. Urethral disruption injuries typically occur in conjunction with multisystem trauma from vehicular accident, falls, or industrial accident. Because the posterior urethra is fixed at both the urogenital diaphragm and the puboprostatic ligaments, the bulbomembranous junction is more vulnerable to injury during pelvic fractures. When the fracture occur the two separated ends fill with scar tissue, resulting in a complete lack of urethral continuity. The location of urethral strictures was classified as penile(including navicularis fossa) , bulbar or posterior (excluding bladder neck contractures).While posterior urethral strictures were commonly caused by traumatic disruption distinctly different from etiology compared to that of anterior strictures disease, recurrence was monitored with the same procedure used for surveillance of anterior urethral reconstruction.

The Urethral disruption is heralded by the triad of blood at the meatus, inability to urinate, and palpably full bladder. When blood at the urethral meatus is discovered, an immediate retrograde urethrogram should be performed to rule out urethral injury.When urethral stricture is diagnosed immediate suprapubic tube placement remains the standard of care.

While the diagnosis of hypospadias needs no radiologic tests, diagnosis of urethral stricture is a matter of discussion. The most common primary diagnostic tests are uroflowmetry (56%), urethrography (51%) and cystourethroscopy (21%). Definition of recurrence of stricture or failure of surgery is also a questionable issue. In 75% of papers regarding urethroplasty, recurrence was defined as the need for additional surgical procedure and in 52% as the need for additional urethral dilation.

The treatment of urethral strictures is divided in two groups; endoscopic and open surgery. The endoscopic treatment such as direct-vision internal urethrotomy are the best reserved for selected short urethral stricture. However when the defects are 1 cm or longer or when a significant corpus spongiofibrosis is present , endoscopic procedure such as cutting through the pelvic scare"cut-to-light" are ineffective. Despite the popularity of this procedure the failure rate after initial urethrotomy is reported to be at least 50%. The failure rate after the second urethrotomy is considered much higher and can be as high as 100%. Therefore there has been continuing discussion about the most appropriate use of urethrotomy, dilation, stenting, and intermittent self dilation. Question have also surfaced about the best technique for urethrotomy. There is no compelling evidence in the literature that any particular form of urethrotomy is more effective than another, whether using a cold knife or laser.

The second treatment option is open surgical reconstruction. There are two kinds of open surgical techniques used for urethroplasty; anastomotic urethroplasty and substitution urethroplasty. Anastomotic urethroplasty involves excision of the strictures and primary anastomosis of urethral ends. Open posterior urethroplasty through a perineal anastomotic approach is the treatment of choice for the most urethral distraction injuries because it definitely cure the patient without the need for multiple procedure. Care must be taken to carefully and meticulously excise all fibrotic tissue from the proximal urethra margin until at least a 28 french bougie passes without resistance. Free tension end to end anastomosis is the procedure of choice when the scar is 1.5-2 cm long and this is highly successful procedure in more than 95% of cases. Urethroplasty remains the gold standard for the management of urethral stricture offering the lowest rate of stricture recurrence and in some circumstance the most cost-effective compared to repeat dilation or endoscopic incision. The limiting factors with anastomotic urethroplasty is the strictures length, in particular the length of component distal to bulbopenile junction. Anastomatic procedure in the bulbar urethra resulted in a significant impairment of erectile function initially which improved in the majority of cases with a low of long term erectile dysfunction.

The second kind of urethroplasty is substitution urethroplasty. Recent advances in tissue graft sources and the introduction of tissue sealants improve surgical outcomes and minimize patients morbidity by decreasing the number of surgical procedures and the potential disfigurement related to graft site morbidity. Substitution urethroplasty can be performed as a one-stage procedure via an augmented anastomotic procedure, patch substitution (onlay procedure) or a circumferential patch, or two-stage procedure which involves the formation of a roof strip followed be second stage tubularization. It has been shown that the efficacy of both grafts and flaps was identical , but there was a much higher morbidity with penile skin flaps which were also more complex with higher morbidity. The graft which has been used included scrotal skin, oral mucosa, extragenital skin, bladder mucosa, and colonic mucosa. The success rate at average follow-up of 53 months was reported to be 60% for augmented anastomotic repair and 80% for onlay procedure.

In conclusion urethroplasty especially in patients with urethral stricture required the urologist to be aware of the techniques which offer the patient the best success. Therefore different considerations have to be taken into account like length , location, anatomy and etiology of stricture. In comparison to reconstruction of urethral stricture, urethroplasty done due to hypospadias seems to be less complicated with high success rate at long term follow-up.

2. Urethral stricture

The bulbous urethra is eccentrically placed in relation to urethra to the corpus spongiosum and much closer to the dorsum of the penile structures. As one moves distally, the pendulous or penile urethra becomes more centrally placed within the corpus spongiousm. Any process that injuries the urethral epithelium or the underlining corpus spongiousm to the point that healing results in a scar an anterior urethral stricture. Today, most urethral stricture are the results of trauma (usually straddle trauma). Inflammatory strictures associated with gonorrhea were the most commonly seen in the past and are less common now due to the effective antibiotic treatment. The place of Chlamydia and Ureaplasma urealyticum (non-specific urethritis) in the development of anterior urethral stricture is not clear. To date, no clear association between nonspecific urethritis and the development of anterior urethral stricture has been established. Congenital stricture is used by some to define a stricture for which there is no identifiable cause. We propose, however to define a stricture as congenital only if it is not an inflammatory stricture, it is a short-length stricture and it is not associated with history of or potential for urethral trauma. And it is the rarest encountered. The location of urethral stricture was classified as penile (including navicularis fossa), bulbar or posterior(excluding bladder neck contracture). According to world health organization posterior urethral stricture are not included in the common definition of urethral stricture and the term stricture is limited to the anterior urethra. Posterior urethral stricture commonly caused by traumatic disruption in contrast to that of anterior stricture.

Beside urethral stricture, congenital anomalies of urethra mandate reconstructive surgery for urethra. Hypospadias is the most common of these causes. Although the definite cause of hypospadias is still undefined, the management of these patients is the same regardless to etiologies or kinds of hypospadias. There are many classification systems for hypospadias depending on the location of the meatus; coronal, subcoronal, midshaft and penoscrotal hypospadias. Hypospadias is seen in approximately 8.2 per 1000 birth [1]. There are more than 200 named surgical procedures for correction of hypospadias with a few common general concept. The aim of hypospadias reconstruction are to achieve an excellent cosmetic result of the penis and to remove chordee to allow for normal sexual intercourse. Tubularized incised plate (TIP) urethroplasty has gained widespread acceptance for repairing hypospadias and has become the therapy of choice for many kinds of hypospadias [2,3,4,5,6]. Tubularized incised urethroplasty was introduced by Snodgrass in 1994, for coronal and subcoronal (distal) cases of hypospadias [3]. Latter on a lot of papers tested the validity of this technique for more complicated hypospadias i.e midshaft and penoscrotal hypospadias and we were from those who claimed such validity [7]. The superiority of TIP urethroplasty technique comes from few key points, midline incision by which the urethral plate is widened to create tension free neourethra, subcutaneous flap which reinforced the neourethra and decrease incidence of fistula (Figure 1 a,b,c,d).

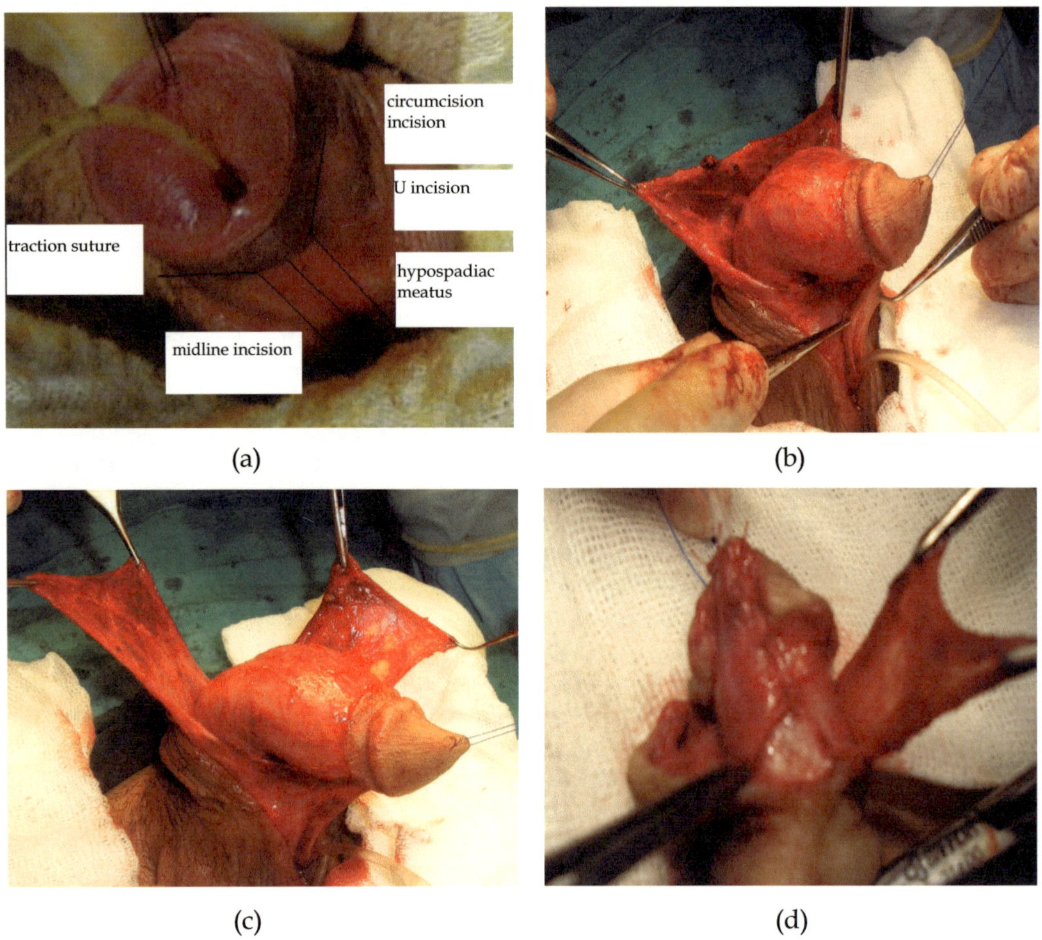

Fig. 1. (a) A 17-year-old patient with penoscrotal hypospadiac meatus where the the main key points of TIP urethroplasty are demonstrated; U-shaped insicion, midline incision in urethroplate, (b) Posterior dartos flap prepared from subcutanous tissue, (c) Dorsal dartos flap is incised from the middle thus both of layer can be rotated ventrally, (d) Shows how both of the layers of the flap covered the neourethra

The most common complication seen in hypospadias correction is urethrocutanous fistula [8,9,10,11]. The rate of fistula was reported to be 3.5% in the present series [12,13]. Several modifications have been introduced on TIP urethroplasty to decrease the rate of fistula, especially regarding the usage of the dorsal dartos flap and we are from the first who applied this novel modification [6,14] (Figure 1). We introduced the usage of double layers dartos flap for the neourethra instead of one layer covering (Figure 1). There were different techniques concerning one layer covering. Retik and Borer described covering the neourethra with an asymmetric rotational subcutaneous dartos tissue flap [15], Yer-kes et al used a Y-to-I warp spongiosum for neourethra reinforcement [16]. Sozubir and Snodgrass [17] also used a dorsal dartos pedicle flap obtained from dorsal prepuce with buttonhole maneuver transposition of flap.

Urethral stricture differed from hypospadias in terms of; etiology, diagnosis, management, success rate and postoperative follow up. The etiology of hypospadias is congenital, however in urethral stricture, wide range of causes are present, traumatic, infectious and congenital cause as we mentioned before. While the physical examination is enough to diagnose hypospadias, the diagnosis of urethral stricture is not so much simple(we will discuss this issue in the coming sections). The surgical management of hypospadias is more simple and lead to more success in comparison to urethroplasty done due to urethral stricture. We will discuss in detail the surgical treatment of urethral stricture.

Urethral stricture refer to anterior urethral disease scaring process involving the spongy erectile tissue of the corpus spongiosum. According to world health organization posterior urethral stricture are not included in the common definition of urethral stricture and the term stricture is limited to the anterior urethra. Because the posterior urethra is fixed at both the urogenital diaphragm and the puboprostatic ligaments, the bulbomembranous junction is more vulnerable to injury during pelvic fracture. In children, injuries are more likely to extend proximally to the bladder because of the rudimentary nature of the prostate.

Diagnosis of urethral stricture begins by physical examination, the triad of blood at urethral meatus, inability to urinate, and palpably full bladder. Urethral disruption is often first detected when urethral catheter cannot be placed or when it is misplaced into pelvic hematoma. Females with urethral injuries presents with vulvar edema and blood at the vaginal introitus, thus indicating the need for careful vaginal examination in all female patients with pelvic fracture. Retrograde Urethrography (RGU) should be done when the blood at urethral meatus is discovered. Small-bore urethral catheter (16 French) is placed unlibricated 1 cm into the fossa navicularis and the balloon is filled with 1 cm of water or Brodney clamp or rolled gauze bandage can be used to provide penile traction. Regarding the usage of local anesthetic jel during retrograde urethrography, recently we published study regarding the usage lidocaine and we concluded that although usage of local anesthetic jel may lead to statistically significant dilatation of urethral diameter, clinically no false negative results in the diagnosis of urethral stricture were observered. [18]. Patients should be placed in an oblique or lateral decubitus position, and it is preferable to perform the study under fluorography, 28 ml of contrast material is injected gently by a 60-ml catheter-tip syringe and the film is taking during injection. The sensitivity and specificity to identify stricture by RGU are 67% to 100% and 93% to 97% with positive and negative predictive values of 50% and 97% to 100% respectively for anterior urethral stricture 3 to 5 cm long [19]. Limitation of RUG and VCUG include readily available fluoroscopic equipment and radiation exposure(1.1 mSV average for VCUG ie equivalent to approximately 11 chest x-rays [20]. Antegrade urethrography can be performed through suprapubic tube placed after reconstruction. The initial management after the immediate diagnosis of urethral trauma is suprapubic catheter. The preoperative evaluation of urethral stricture before reconstructive procedure is planned, are imaging studies are necessary to delineate the characteristics of urethral stricture defect. A cystogram and retrograde urethrogram should be obtained simultaneously. Besides these mains method of diagnosis a lot of methods can help in detecting urethral stricture; voiding symptoms and questionnaires described in the clinical history of the patient is the most basic and essential screening procedure to detect stricture. Multiple studies have evaluated the correlation between the AUA-SS and the presence of urethral stricture. The AUA-SS has been inversely correlated with urethral diameters by retrograde urethrogram and flow rates by uroflowmetry [21] .Morey et al demonstrated significant improvement in AUA-SS after successful urethroplasty that correlated with radiographic evidence of a patent urethra by retrograde urethrogram in 41of 50 patients [22]. Urine culture/ urinary tract infection occurred due to increased post-void residual (PVR) and urinary stasis in patients with stricture. Urinary tract infection (UTI) is a common complication immediately after urethroplasty at reported rate of 6% [23]. To our knowledge no study has correlated postoperative UTI with stricture recurrence. Further studies are needed to determine the usefulness of urine culture as screening methods and the correlation between symptomatic UTI and stricture recurrence. Ultrasound PVR measurement is noninvasive technique that provide objective measurement of bladder emptying [24]. One may predict that high PVR volume would predict stricture. Unfortunately sonographic measurement are often user dependent with high interest variability [25] and up to two-third of patients may demonstrate daily variability in PVR of greater than 600m [26]. Uroflowmetry is one of the most used measures to evaluate stricture. It is easily performed noninvasive and may allow quantitive data regarding voiding patterns[27]. Similar to ultrasound PVR, flow rates may be affected by operator error, benign prostate hyperplasia (BPH), lower urinary tract symptom, bladder dysfunction and variation in bladder capacity [28]. Further limitation of uroflowmetry include the needed for a minimum voided volume of 125 to 150 ml to reach a voided flow rate that reliably predicts an abnormality. Urethral ultrasound is relatively new technique for the evaluation of urethral stricture disease. First described by the McAninch et al in 1988 [29], urethral ultrasound(UU) to identify stricture has a reported sensitivity of 66% to 100%, specificity of 97% to 98%, and positive and negative predictive values of 50% to 80% and 96% to 98% respectively for anterior stricture 3 to 5 cm long. The usefulness of UU is limited by stricture location as it is more sensitive to stricture in the penile urethra than in bulbar portion [30]. It is also user dependency and the semi-invasive nature of the procedure often requiring local or general anesthesia for full urethra distention. It is benefit it can give three dimensional information about the stricture location and length. Magnetic resonance (MR) urethrography is a promising tool for defining male urethral strictures. It has comparable results with the combined RUG and SUG in diagnosing the anterior and posterior urethral strictures as regard the site and extension and degree of spongiofibrosis but MR is superior in diagnosis of associated pathologies with stricture as it can provide extra-guidance for treatment planning that cannot be obtained with RUG [31,32].

In one of the most large systematic review for the diagnosis for recurrence stricture recurrence after urethroplasty conducted by Meeks et al [33] in their analysis of urethroplasty publication since 2000 found urethroplasty outcomes was determined by up to eight different diagnostics tests. The most common were uroflowmetry 56%,and retrograde urethrography 51%. Cystourethrography was used in 25% of patients. Recurrence of stricture was defined as the need for an additional surgical procedure or dilatation in 75% and 52% of articles respectively . Clearly standardization is required and the methods used to determine stricture recurrence after urethroplasty remain widely variable. There are many objective and subjective procedures to evaluate for stricture recurrence. Standardization of A surveillance protocol after urethroplasty is needed to more effectively compare outcomes among institutions.

In our opinion both objective and subjective patients satisfaction outcomes should be evaluated. Objective measures should be ideally involve urethrography or cystourethroscopy, flow rate is a poor indicator of urethral lumen diameters and a significant impact on flow rate is not obververed until the urethral diameters is below 11F.

3. Treatment of urethral stricture; Endoscopic or open surgery?

3.1 Endoscopic management

The management of urethral stricture disease in adult males has a wide range of possible therapeutics treatments. Urethral stricture are often treated with urethrotomy most commonly direct vision internal urethrotomy (DVIU) [34,35]. The popularity of this procedure has been attributed to the ease of performance, a perceived low complication rate and the fact that many north American urologists don not perform open urethroplasty so they may be forced to perform repeat urethrotomy[34,36]. The failure after initial urethrotomy is reported to be 50% [37,38]. The failure after second urethrotomy is considered much higher and can be as high as 100% [35,37,38]. Santucci R et al [39] performed retrospective review of more than 100 patients as a first study in north America, to evaluate the stricture free rate not only after single urethrotomy but after 2 through 5 procedure. He concluded that urethrotomy is a popular treatment for male urethral stricture. However the performance characteristics are poor. The Success rates after 1 urethrotomy was a mere 8% and after multiple urethrotomies was close to 0%. Because urethroplasty has long-term success rate ranging from 75-100 , increased use of this more effective treatment may be warranted[40]. Urethrotmoy should be reserved as a temporizing measure for poor surgical candidates until further reconstruction can be planned and executed. The majority of the base evidence base for the management of urethral strictures dos not reach level 1 according to the oxford classification. With the rarity of significantly powered randomized controlled trials, we have to look to observational studies and expert opinion for guidance. In recent years there has been continuing discussion about the most appropriate use of urethrotomy, dilatation, stenting and intermittent self dilatation. We believe that self intermittent dilatation may be beneficial at least in prolonging the period between urethrotomies. There is no compelling evidence in literature that any particular from of urethrotomy is more effective than another, whether using a cold knife or laser. Heyns et al looked at whether repeated dilatation or urethrotomy was useful and noted that after single treatment 70% would be stricture free at three months, 35-40% would be remain stricture free at 24 months, but not at 48 months. A third treatment was of no benefit at all [41].

Successful out comes from urethrotomy or dilatation requires adequate vascularity within the under lining corpus spongiusom and is more likely to be successful in the bulbar urethra. Whilest et al [42] found up to two internal urethrotomy did not affect the outcomes or likelihood of subsequent anastomotic urethroplasty in patients with posterior injuries. For the anterior urethra using cox hazards regression analysis, failed internal urethrotomy

has been found to conform increased risk of failure for consequent urethroplasty [43]. Morey concluded that carful preoperative evaluation should be undertaken prior to internal urethrotomy and a patient should not need to have failed minimally invasive therapy prior to being considered for urethroplasty [44]. The current evidence suggests that the success is dependent upon stricture position, cause and length with success decline as the length of the stricture increases as clearly demonstrated by heyns et al [41]. Altaf et al reported that one attempt at direct vision internal urethrotomy can be considered in the most bulbar stricture, unless they are complicated. For example by previous open surgery or fistulae, whilst a primary urethroplasty may be more appropriate in penile stricture [45]. This algorithm of considering an initial urethrotomy has been also been reiterated by Wessells to be the most cost effective [46]. Injection of triamcinolone (antifibroblast and anticollagen properties) was submucosally in 25 patients undergoing urethroplasty, reduced recurrence rates to 21.7% as compared to 50% in a control group at one year [47]. All the patients had stricture less than 1.5 cm and the author randomized the treatment with no mention of blinding.
Stents were introduced a number of years ago but unfortunately have not stayed the test of time since they have been clearly shown to be associated with complications [48]. Particularly if they are inserted as management of the a failed urethroplasty following a urethral distraction injuries [49]. Failure of a permanently implanted urethral stent represents a significant therapeutic challenge which often leads to difficult substitution procedure with consequent limitation of the success of the procedure [49,50]. Therefore usage of stent should be limited to exceptional cases i.e difficult recalcitrant posterior urethral stenosis [51].

3.2 Open surgical techniques

The second treatment option is open surgical techniques or urethroplasty. Urethroplasty remain the most effective therapy for the management of most cases of anterior urethral stricture. Anastomatic urethroplasty involves excision of the stricture and the primary anastomosis of urethral ends. Traditionally strictures up to 3 cm have been considered as suitable for primary anastomosis. The limiting factors with anastomotic urethroplasty is the stricture length, in particular the length of the component distal to the bulbopenile junction. Open posterior urethroplasty through a perineal anastomotic approach is the treatment of choice for the most urethral distraction injuries because it definitely cure the patients without the need for multiple surgeries. One must be caution of the risk of penile curvature and shortening, so mobilization of the urethra must not encroach upon the penile urethra. For bulbar stricture, by freeing up the urethra from the corpora and separating the two corpora another few centimeters may be gained in length depending on the individual circumstances. If the anastomotic urethroplasty is possible it is the procedure of choice having a success rate of approximately 90% at the intermediate follow-up [52,53]. In the patients with a 2-5 cm stricture undergoing an anastomotic procedure the risk erectile dysfunction is increased [54]. A prospective study of erectile function posturethroplasty showed anastomotic procedure in the bulbar urethra resulted in a significant impairment of erectile function initially which improved in the majority of cases. With low risk of long-term [55].
Substitution urethroplasty; this technique can be performed as one stage procedure via an augmented anastomotic procedure, (patch substitution onlay procedure) or a circumferential patch, or two stage procedure which involves the formation of a roof strip followed by second-stage tubularization. Balbagli and colleagues [56] reported their results in using

dorsal onlay graft urethroplasty and reported a series of 38 patients in which 65.8% were considered successful over a mean follow up of 111 months. The majority of the recurrence in this study occurred in the first year. Certainly in the long term follow up it is clear that the recurrence rate after a substitution is far worse than many would otherwise have considered likely based on the existing literature, with a reported rate of 42% at 15 years for substitution procedure and 14% for anastomotic procedure [57]. Barbagli et al [53] analyzed a cohort of 375 patients who underwent one of the three different one –stage procedure for bulbar strictures. He found that at an average follow up of 53 months the success rate for anastomotic urethroplasty was 90.9% and the augmented anastomotic repair was 60% and the onlay procedure was 80%. The Asopa technique, involving dorsal placement of a buccal mucosal graft via a ventral approach, has also been evaluated with 87% success rate at mean follow up of 42 months [58]. Another group found better success rate when applying a dorsal lingual mucosal graft via a ventral urethrotomy approach than a conventional barbagli approach of urethral mobilization [59]. However the preoperative characteristics of the patients in the group that underwent the balbagli approach include patients with higher proportion of patients with pan-urethral disease and balanitis Xerotica obliterans /infective causes potentially confounding interpretation of the results. Kulkarni et al have interestingly described better success rat with a one two stage oral mucosal urethroplasty 91 vs 73% respectively for penile stricture associated with lichen sclerosis [60]. However the number of the cases was low 8 and 15 respectively also the follow up period was short thus its difficult to draw any definite conclusion. Recently Kulkarini et al [61] have described the use of the one-sided anterior urethroplasry utilizing oral mucosa to preserve the lateral vascular supply to the urethra. Of 24 patients 92% had a successful outcomes at the mean of 22 months follow up. However the preservation of the lateral vascular supply of the urethra is of clinical values or not is still under debate. Barbagli et al [62] described a step to spare the bulbospongiosus nerves and muscles when gaining access for urethroplasty in series of sex patients. In all sex patients no evidence of stricture recurrence was noted at 12 months.

Type of the grafts which have been used include scrotal skin [63], extragenital skin [64] and bladder mucosa [65]. In contemporary practice genital skin or oral mucosa are the most used, although there is interest in the future in the potential for tissue engineering [66]. Genital skin is flap are particularly useful when dealing with stricture in the penile urethra when an onlay flap of penile skin can be particularly helpful. Oral mucosa was first described in 1941 by Humby and Higgins [67]. This mucosa is used to being wet and is resilient to skin diseases such as lichen sclerosis and has a privileged immunology. Barbagli et al [68] in their retrospective review of 350 patients undergoing oral mucosa harvest from a single check showed the majority of patients had no pain 85.2% or major complication. Mathur et al [69] described the successful use of the tunica albugina from the corpora for the urethroplasty with re-operation rate of 9.2% at 3 years in 206 patients . In 36 cases ranging between 10 and 20 cm in length, Xu et al [70] described success rates of 85.7% at a mean of 53.6 months using colonic mucosa . Similarly Munday and Andrich [71] described the use of grafts from the stomach, ileum and colon in complex patients with bulbomembranous strictures showing some success in otherwise unsalvageable cases. Tissue-engineering grafts of urethra offers a promising alternative to current grafts and minimize the risk of donor site morbidity [72]. A cellular grafts have undergone clinical assessment with mixed results [73,74]. Contemporary work is concentrated upon developing a cellular tissue engineered graft and Li et al [75] have shown a reduced inflammatory response and no recurrence of stricture up to 6 months in a rabbit model. Lu at al [76] have reported on the in-vitro success of culturing urothelial cells on a cellular bladder matrix making the cellular graft histologically like urothelium.

In the future and in order to aid the decision-making process for the managements of stricture disease, randomized controlled studies (RCT) should be conducted [77,78]. Most of the current evidence comes from observational studies and due to the low qualities of cases available for RCT selection numbers are often increased by widening the inclusion criteria and thus comparing cases of different causes, locations and strictures size. It is clear that a more homogenous patients selection may guide clinical decisions better. Many factors have been found to affect urethroplasty outcomes and should thus be accounted for preoperatively [43,79]. Moreover, it must be noted that although evidence may support one technique over another, the situation during urethroplasty requires a dynamics assessment and adoption of an achievable procedure leading to patient-centered success.

4. Conclusion

The plastic surgery of urethra include wide range of indications, operative techniques and outcomes. Urethroplasty done due to hypospadias is of more success rates in comparison to urethroplasty done due to urethral strictures. The surgeons have consensus on the preferable technique for hypospadias repair, however the situation is not similar regarding the management of urethral strictures. The contemporary evidence for the management of urethral strictures provides a practice-based algorithm which a reconstructive urologist may utilize when dealing with strictures based on location, length, anatomy and etiology. Moreover every case is unique and often different consideration have to be taken into account in carrying out surgery , with urologist being aware of the entire armamentarium of techniques and needing to use them to provide the best result for each patient. Therefore we believe that there is a need for a multi-center international database with outcomes standardization to adequately develop higher levels of comparative evidence. The development of validate patient-reported outcome measures is going to be very important in achieving this goal.

5. References

[1] Sweet RA, Schortt HG, Kurland R et al. Study of incidence of hypospadias in Rochester, Minnesota 1940-1970 and a case control comparison of possible etiologic factors. Mayo Clin Proc 1974; 49: 52.

[2] Snodgrass W, Koyle M, Manzoni G et al. Tubularized incised plate hypospadias repair for proximal hypospadias. J Urol 1998; 159:2129-2131.

[3] Sondgrass W. Tubularized incised plate urethroplasty for distal hypospadias. J Urol 1994; 151:464-465.

[4] Sondgrass W, Koyle M, Manzoni G et al. Tabularized incised plate for hypospadias repair: result of a multicenter experience. J Urol 1996; 156:839-841.

[5] Sondgrass WT, Lorenzo A. Tubularized incised plate urethroplasty for hypospadias reoperation. Br J Urol Int 2002; 89:98-100.

[6] Mustafa M, Wadie BS, Abol-Enein H. Standard Snodgrass technique in conjunction with double-layer covering of the neourethra with dorsal dartos flap is the therapy of first choice for hypospadias.. Int Urol Nephrol. 2008; 40(3):573-6.

[7] Mustafa M.The concept of tubularized incised plate hypospadias repair for different types of hypospadias.Int Urol Nephrol. 2005; 37(1):89-91.
[8] Sugarman ID,Trevett J, Malone PS. Tubularization of the incised plate(Snodgrass procedure) for the primary hypospadias surgery. BJU Int 1999; 83:88-90.
[9] Jayanthi VR. The modified Snodgrass hypospadias repair: reducing the risk of fistula and meatal stenosis J Urol 2003; 170:1603-1605.
[10] Djordjevic ML, Perovic SV, Slavkovic Z, Djarovic N: longitudinal dorsal dartos flap for preventing of fistula after a Snodgrass hypospadias. Eur Urol 2006; 53-57.
[11] Djordjevic ML, Perovic SV, Vukadinovic VM: Dorsal dartos flap for preventing fistula in the Snodgrass hypospadias repair. BJU Int 2005; 95:1303-1309.
[12] Sondgrass W: Tubularized incised plate urethroplasty for distal hypospadias. J Urol 1994:151:464-465.
[13] Sondgrass W, Koyle M, Manzoni G, et al: Tubularized incised plate for hypospadias repair : result of a multicenter experience. J Urol 1996; 156:839-841.
[14] Mustafa M, Wadie BS, Abol-Enein H . Dorsal dartos flap in Snodgrass hypospadias repair: how to use it?.Urol Int. 2008; 81(2):215-7.
[15] Retik A B, Borer JG: Primary and reoperative hypospadias repair with the Snodgrass technique. World J Urol 1998; 16:186-191.
[16] Yerkes EB, Adams MC, Miller DA, Pope JC, Rink RC, Brock JW 3rd: Y-to-I warp: use of the distal spongiosum for hypospadias repair. J Urol 2000; 163:1536-1539.
[17] Sozubir S, Snodgrass W: A new algorithm for primary hypospadias repair based on TIP urethroplasty. J Pediatr Surg 2003; 38:1157-1161.
[18] Mustafa M, Ali-El-Dein B, Mohsen T, Ibrahiem el-HI.The use of local anesthetic gel during retrograde urethrography: does it cause a false negative result? Int Urol Nephrol. 2007; 39(2):513-6.
[19] Choudhary S, Singh P, Sundar E et al: A comparison of sonourethrography and retrograde urethrography in evaluation of anterior urethral strictures. Clin Radiol 2004; 59: 736.
[20] Arbique 13M, 13illeran JP, 13uild JB et al: Radiation exposure during standing voiding cystourethrography in women. Urology 2006; 67: 269.
[21] Heyns CF and Marais DC: Prospective evaluation of the American Urological Association symptom index and peak urinary flow rate for the followup of men with known urethral stricture disease. J Urol 2002; 168: 2051.
[22] Morey AF, McAninch JW, Duckett CP et al: American UrologicalAssociation symptom index in the assessment of urethroplasty outcomes. J Urol1998; 159: 1192.
[23] Navai N, Erickson BA, Zhao LC et al: Complications following urethral reconstructive surgery: a six year experience. Int Braz J Urol 2008; 34: 594.
[24] Kaplan SA, Wein AJ, Staskin DR et al: Urinary retention and post-void residual urine in men: separating truth from tradition. J Urol 2008; 180: 47.
[25] Rule AD, Jacobson DJ, Mc13ree ME et al: Longitudinal changes in post-void residual and voided volume among community dwelling men. J Urol 2005; 174: 1317.
[26] Dunsmuir WD, Feneley M, Corry DA et al: The day-to-day variation (test-retest reliability) of residualurine measurement. Br J Urol 1996; 77: 192.
[27] Feneley MR, Dunsmuir WD, Pearce J et al: Reproducibility of uroflow measurement: experience during a double-blind, placebo-controlled study of doxazosin in benign prostatic hyperplasia. Urology 1996; 47: 658.

[28] Colomb J, Lindner A, Siegel Y et al: Variability and circadian changes in home uroflowmetry in patients with benign prostatic hyperplasia compared to normalcontrols. J Urol 1992; 147: 1044.
[29] McAninch JW, Laing FC and Jeffrey RB Jr: Sonourethrography in the evaluation of urethral strictures: a preliminary report. J Urol 1988; 139: 294.
[30] Nash PA, McAninch JW, Bruce JE et al: Sonourethrography in the evaluation of anterior urethral strictures. J Urol 1995; 154: 72.
[31] Osman Y, El-Ghar MA, Mansour O, Refaie H, El-Diasty T. Magnetic resonance urethrography in comparison to retrograde urethrography in diagnosis of male urethral strictures: is it clinically relevant? Eur Urol. 2006; 50(3):587-93.
[32] El-Ghar MA, Osman Y, Elbaz E, Refiae H, El-Diasty T. MR urethrogram versus combined retrograde urethrogram and sonourethrography in diagnosis of urethral stricture . Eur J Radiol.2010; 74(3):193-8.
[33] Meeks JJ, Erickson BA, Granieri MA, Gonzalez CM. Stricture recurrence after urethroplasty:a systematic review. J Urol 2009; 182:1266–1270.
[34] Greenwell TJ, Castle C, Andrich DE et al: Repeat urethrotomy and dilation for the treatment of urethral stricture are neither clinically effective not cost-effective. J Urol 2004; 172: 275.
[35] Naude AM and Heyns CF: What is the place of internal urethrotomy in the treatment of urethral stricture disease? Nat Clin Pract Urol 2005; 2: 538.
[36] Bullock TL and Brandes SB: Adult anterior urethral strictures: a national practice patterns survey of board certified urologists in the United States. J Urol 2007; 177: 685.
[37] Heyns CF, Steenkamp JW, De Kock ML et al: Treatment of male urethral strictures: is repeated dilation or internal urethrotomy useful? J Urol 1998; 160: 356.
[38] Pansadoro V and Emiliozzi P: Internal urethrotomy in the management of anterior urethral strictures: long-term followup. J Urol 1996; 156: 73.
[39] Santucci R., Eisenberg L: Urethrotomy has a much lower success rate than previously reported. J Urol 2010; 183:1859-1862.
[40] Santucci RA: Male urethral stricture disease. In: Urologic Diseases in America. Edited by MS Litwin and CS Saigal. US Department of Health and Human Services, Public Health Service, National Institutes of Health, National Institute of Diabetes and Digestive and Kidney Diseases. Washington, D.C.: US Government Publishing Office 2007; NIH publication No. 07-5512, pp 531–552.
[41] Heyns CF, Steenkamp JW, de Kock ML, Whitaker P. Treatment of male urethral strictures: is repeated dilation or internal urethrotomy useful? J Urol 1998; 160:356–358.
[42] Singh BP, Andankar MG, Swain SK, et al. Impact of prior urethral manipulation on outcome of anastomotic urethroplasty for posttraumatic urethral stricture. Urology 2009; 75:179–182.
[43] Breyer BN, McAninch JW, Whitson JM, et al. Multivariate analysis of risk factors for long-term urethroplasty outcome. J Urol 2009; 183:613–617.
[44] Morey A. Urethral stricture is now an open surgical disease. J Urol 2009; 181 :953–954.
[45] Mangera A, Christopher C. Management of anterior urethral stricture: an evidence-based approach. Current opinion in urology 2010; 20:453-458.

[46] Wessells H. Cost-effective approach to short bulbar urethral strictures supports single internal urethrotomy before urethroplasty. J Urol 2009; 181:954- 955.
[47] Mazdak H, Izadpanahi MH, Ghalamkari A, et al. Internal urethrotomy and intraurethral submucosal injection of triamcinolone in short bulbar urethral strictures. Int Urol Nephrol 2009.
[48] Hussain M, Greenwell TJ, Shah J, Mundy A. Long-term results of a self-expanding wallstent in the treatment of urethral stricture. BJU Int 2004; 94:1037-1039.
[49] Chapple CR, Bhargava S. Management of the failure of a permanently implanted urethral stent-a therapeutic challenge. Eur Urol 2008; 54:665- 670.
[50] Palminteri E, Gacci M, Berdondini E, etal. Management of urethral stent failure for recurrent anterior urethral strictures. Eur Urol 2010; 57:615-21.
[51] Eisenberg ML, Elliott SP, McAninch JW. Preservation of lower urinary tract function in posterior urethral stenosis: selection of appropriate patients for urethral stents. J Urol 2007; 178:2456–2460.
[52] Lumen N, Piet H, Willem O. Urethroplasty for urethral strictures: quality assessment of an in-home algorithm. Int J Urol 2010; 17:167–174.
[53] Barbagli G, Guazzoni G, Lazzeri M. One-stage bulbar urethroplasty: retrospective analysis of the results in 375 patients. Eur Urol 2008; 53:828–833.
[54] Xie H, Xu YM, Xu XL, et al. Evaluation of erectile function after urethral reconstruction: a prospective study. Asian J Androl 2009; 11:209–214.
[55] Erickson BA, Granieri MA, Meeks JJ, et al. Prospective analysis of erectile dysfunction after anterior urethroplasty:incidence and recovery of function. J Urol 2010; 183:657–661.
[56] Barbagli G, Morgia G, Lazzeri M. Dorsal onlay skin graft bulbar urethroplasty: long-term follow-up. Eur Urol 2008; 53:628–633.
[57] Andrich DE, Dunglison N, Greenwell TJ, Mundy AR. The long-term results of urethroplasty. J Urol 2003; 170:90–92.
[58] Pisapati VL, Paturi S, Bethu S, etal. Dorsal buccal mucosal graft urethroplasty for anterior urethral stricture by Asopa technique. Eur Urol 2009; 56:201 - 205.
[59] Singh PB, Das SK, Kumar A, et al. Dorsal onlay lingual mucosal graft urethroplasty:comparison of two techniques. Int J Urol 2008; 15:1002- 1005.
[60] Barbagli G, De AM, Romano G, Lazzeri M. Clinical outcome and quality of life assessment in patients treated with perineal urethrostomy for anterior urethral stricture disease. J Urol 2009; 182:548–557.
[61] Kulkarni S, Barbagli G, Sansalone S, Lazzeri M. One-sided anterior urethroplasty: a new dorsal onlay graft technique. BJU Int 2009; 104:1150–1155.
[62] Barbagli G, De SS, Annino F, et al. Muscle- and nerve-sparing bulbar urethroplasty:a new technique. Eur Urol 2008; 54:335–343.
[63] Jordan GH. Scrotal and perineal flaps for anterior urethral reconstruction. Urol Clin North Am 2002; 29:411–416.
[64] Vyas PR, Roth DR, Perlmutter AD. Experience with free grafts in urethral reconstruction. J Urol 1987; 137:471 -474.
[65] Xu YM, Qiao Y, Sa YL, et al. Urethral reconstruction using colonic mucosa graft for complex strictures. J Urol 2009; 1 82:1040–1043.
[66] Bhargava S, Patterson JM, Inman RD, et al. Tissue-engineered buccal mucosa urethroplasty-clinical outcomes. Eur Urol 2008; 53:1263–1269.

[67] Humby G, Higgins T. A one-stage operation for hypospadias. Br J Surg 2009; 29:84–92.
[68] Barbagli G, Vallasciani S, Romano G, et al. Morbidity of oral mucosa graft • • harvesting from a single cheek. Eur Urol 2010; 58:33-41.
[69] Mathur RK, Sharma AK, Odiya S. Tunica albuginea urethroplasty for anterior urethral strictures: a urethroscopic analysis. Int J Urol 2009; 16:751 –755.
[70] Xu YM, Qiao Y, Sa YL, et al. Urethral reconstruction using colonic mucosa graft for complex strictures. J Urol 2009; 182:1040–1043.
[71] Mundy AR, Andrich DE. Entero-urethroplasty for the salvage of bulbo-membranous stricture disease or trauma. BJU Int 2009; 105:1716–1720.
[72] Jenkins BJ, Badenoch DF, Fowler CG, Blandy JP. Long-term results of treatment of urethral injuries in males caused by external trauma. Br J Urol 1992; 70:73–75.
[73] El-Kassaby A, Aboushwareb T, Atala A. Randomized comparative study between buccal mucosal and acellular bladder matrix grafts in complex anterior urethral strictures. J Urol 2008; 1 79:1432–1436.
[74] Ecke TH, Hallmann S, Gerullis H, Ruttloff J. Reconstruction of the urethra with a Surgisis onlay patch in urethral reconstructive surgery:two case reports. J Med Case Reports 2009; 3:7232.
[75] Li C, Xu Y, Song L, et al. A preliminary experimental study on urethral reconstruction using tissue engineered oral mucosa. Zhongguo Xiu Fu Chong Jian Wai Ke Za Zhi 2008; 22:1 242–1 245.
[76] Lu MJ, Wang Z, Zhou GD, et al. Construction of urethra mucosa structure in vitro by tissue engineering. Zhonghua Nan Ke Xue 2008; 14:1072–1076.
[77] Barbagli G, Lazzeri M. Can reconstructive urethral surgery proceed without randomized controlled trials? Eur Urol 2008; 54:709–711.
[78] Capizzi A. Urethral surgery in the evidence-based medicine (EBM) era:a never-ending story. Urology 2009; 73:1172–1174.
[79] Breyer BN, McAninch JW, Whitson JM, et al. Effect of obesity on urethroplasty outcome. Urology 2009; 73:1352–1355.

5

Management of Post Hypospadias Urethral Fistula

Sherif Shehata and Mohamed Hashish
Department of Pediatric Surgery, Tanta University Hospital, Tanta, Egypt

1. Introduction

Complications after any surgical procedures are normal consequences within the standard acceptable percentage among surgeons. Complications are higher in hypospadias surgery as compared to other reconstructive operations. Urethrocutaneous fistula after hypospadias surgery repair is the most common complication and remains a frustrating problem for surgeons [21].

Generally fistula is defined as a tract connecting two epithelial surfaces. Furthermore, the problem is exacerbated because urethrocutaneous fistula not only occurs but also recurs, sometimes with all the potential harmful physical and psychological consequences. However, with the improvement in suture material and surgical techniques, such complications are increasingly unacceptable. The occurrence of urethrocutaneous fistulae precludes a goal of hypospadias surgery [6].

The reported incidence of urethrocutaneous fistula ranged, from 0 to 30%, varying with the severity of hypospadias, surgical technique, and experience of the operating surgeon [5]. Unfortunately there is no one single perfect technique to repair any urethrocutaneous fistula. The temptation to simply close the hole without understanding the failure mechanisms is dangerous and often leads to recurrence of the fistula or even worse [29].

Many factors influence the results of fistula repair such as the conditions of local tissue, time after hypospadias repair, the number, location and size of the fistula [29]. These factors can be preventable when considered, experience and surgical tips are needed to improve the outcomes in cases of hypospadias fistulae.

2. Incidence of fistula formation

Generally, the incidence of fistula varies from 0 to 30 %. It is less in urethral plate preservation procedures like tabularized incised plate (TIP) and onlay flap as compared to inner preputial flap and tube urethroplasty.

The incidence of fistula formation has decreased gradually in the past two decades. In 1973, Horton and Devine estimated the incidence of fistula following hypospadias surgery to range between 15 % and 45 % [18]. In 1984, Shapiro found a urethral fistula rate of 6.25 % in a series of 176 hypospadias repairs including various techniques of repair [32].

Nowadays, the incidence of fistula was varied among different techniques of repair as some procedures are more prone to fistula formation than others [15]. For example, Durham

Smith in 1981 noted that the fistula rate for the meatoplasty and glanuloplasty (MAGPI) procedure ranged from 0.5 % to 10 %, whereas the rate for flip-flap repairs varied from 2.2 % to 35 % and that for island pedicle tube repairs from 4 % to 33 % [37]. Free graft tube-repairs are encountered with higher fistula rates of 15-50 %. While using a two-stage repair, in more than 500 cases, Durham Smith in 1990 reduced his incidence of fistula formation to less than 3 % [36]. Similarly, Greenfield and colleagues reported a urethral fistula rate of 2.5 % with a two-stage repair [12].

3. Classification of fistula

The Beginning of fistula formation occurs early in the healing process after ventral urethral repair usually between the 7th-10th post operative days [3].
Post hypospadias urethral fistula could be classified according to many aspects into different classifications:

1. According to site or location into:
   - Anastomotic fistula
   - Non anastomotic fistula

   The urethrocutaneous fistula may occur anywhere along the neourethra. However, the most common sites include the site of the original meatus, glans penis, at the coronal level in tubularization urethroplasty and at the site of anastomosis in flap urethroplasty [8].
2. According to the size into:
   - Pin point fistula
   - Small fistula
   - Mega fistula.

   Small tiny fistulas may occur even with experienced surgeons using delicate techniques. Mega fistula with diameter more than 4-5 mm in its largest diameter represents a form of incomplete disruption of the repair [11].

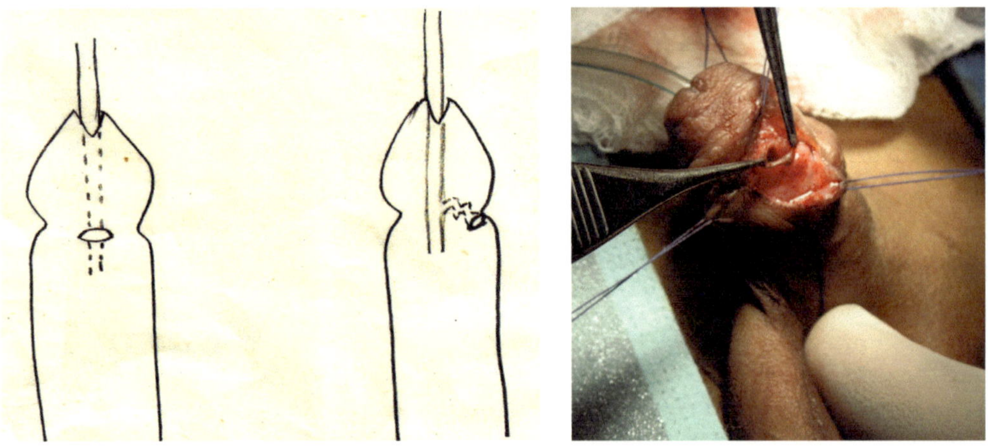

(a) (b) (c)

Fig. 1. Description of some types of fistula according to fistula track path: A) Graph of direct ventral fistula, B) Graph of serpentine long lateral fistula and C) Operative photograph of direct post anastomotic fistula. [Courtesy of Prof. Sherif Shehata]

3. According to its track path into:
   - Direct
   - Serpentine

   Direct fistula where the tract pass straight in the same level of all repaired layers while serpentine fistula where the tract ruin in different pathway among the different layers and usually came lateral in position not in the mid line.
4. According to number into:
   - Single
   - Multiple

   Single fistula are more common and may be presented in different size while the Multiple fistulae are less common; they may occur due to technical factors such as ischemia, infection and distal stenosis or in recurrent cases [11].

4. Mechanism of fistula formation

Infection and ischemia remain the two important factors in fistula production. Incorporation of urethral mucosa in the ventral repair is a substrate for fistula formation with rapid migration of urethral mucosa and skin epithelium into suture tracts. Whether the mucosal or dermal migration along suture tracts can be attenuated or prevented by changing the biochemical environment needs further investigation [7]. Some individuals have abnormal tissue reactivity to the sutures as foreign bodies, thus induce irritation and inflammatory reaction that initiates fistula formation [34].

5. Etiology and risk factors

The actual causes of fistulae formation remain unknown although the most common reasons are technical and avoidable; there are many factors that may cause a high incidence of fistula formation which include:

1. Local infection,
2. Local ischemia,
3. An inadequate procedure,
4. Poor tissue healing, and
5. Distal obstruction due to meatal stenosis/encrustation [24, 34].
6. The type of suture material.

The fistula formation rate was significantly higher in the group of patients where neourethra was constructed using 6/0 polyglactine (Vicryl) in a single layer, full-thickness, uninterrupted fashion (16.6 %) compared to group of patients in which 7/0 polydioxanone (PDS) was used in the urethral anastomosis performed in a subcuticular, uninterrupted fashion with fistula rate of 4.9 % [23, 24]. Use of a subcutaneous suture technique utilizing PDS suture material in urethroplasties is advocated [23, 24].

6. Tips for fistula prevention

The numerous factors that have accounted to lower incidence of fistula formation today are summarized below:

1. Technical points
   - Type of suture
   - Fine instruments

    - Magnification
2. Protective intermediate layer
    - De-epithelialized skin
    - Tunica vaginalis
    - Dartos flap
    - Dorsal subcutaneous preputial flap
    - External spermatic fascia
3. Urethral stenting
4. Dressing
5. Tisseel (fibrin glue) [15]

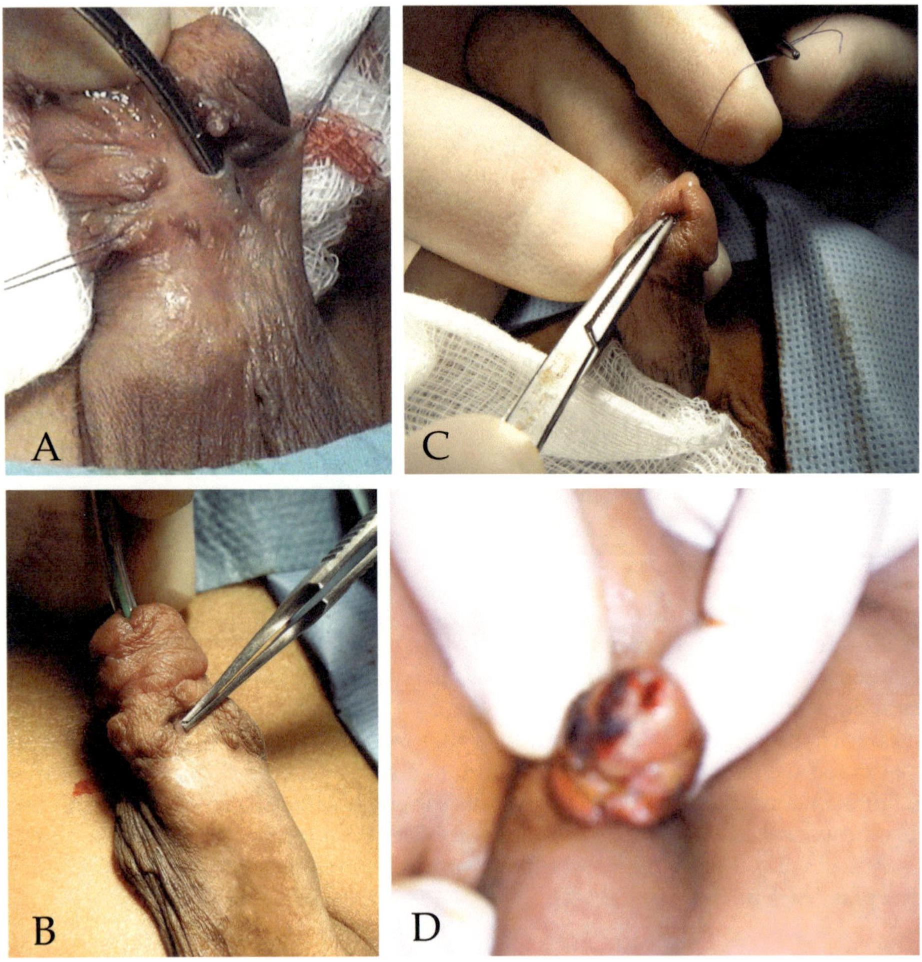

Fig. 2. Shape and Causes of post hypospadias fistulae: A) Preoperative photograph shows disrupted proximal hypospadias with multiple fistulae with operative calibration, B) Operative photograph of a case of direct coronal fistula, C) Photograph of the a case of meatal stenosis as a contributing factor to fistula development and D) Postoperative photograph of another case of distal hypospadias with early infection that predispose to fistula formation later. [Courtesy of Prof. Sherif Shehata]

6.1 Technical points

Better and finer suture materials are available today with greater tensile strength and less reactivity including 6-0 to 7-0 polyglactin (Vicryl) and polyglycolic acid (Dexon). These sutures can be used on the skin as well as internally. PDS should not be used in the urethra (subcuticular is satisfactory) because it may react with urine and fistula may result [9, 23]. Plastic surgical principles such as ophthalmic and microvascular instruments are advocated and delicate tissue handling are now should be used by most hypospadias surgeons. Also most surgeons use either the microscope or 2.5 - 3.5 X optical magnification [9, 30].

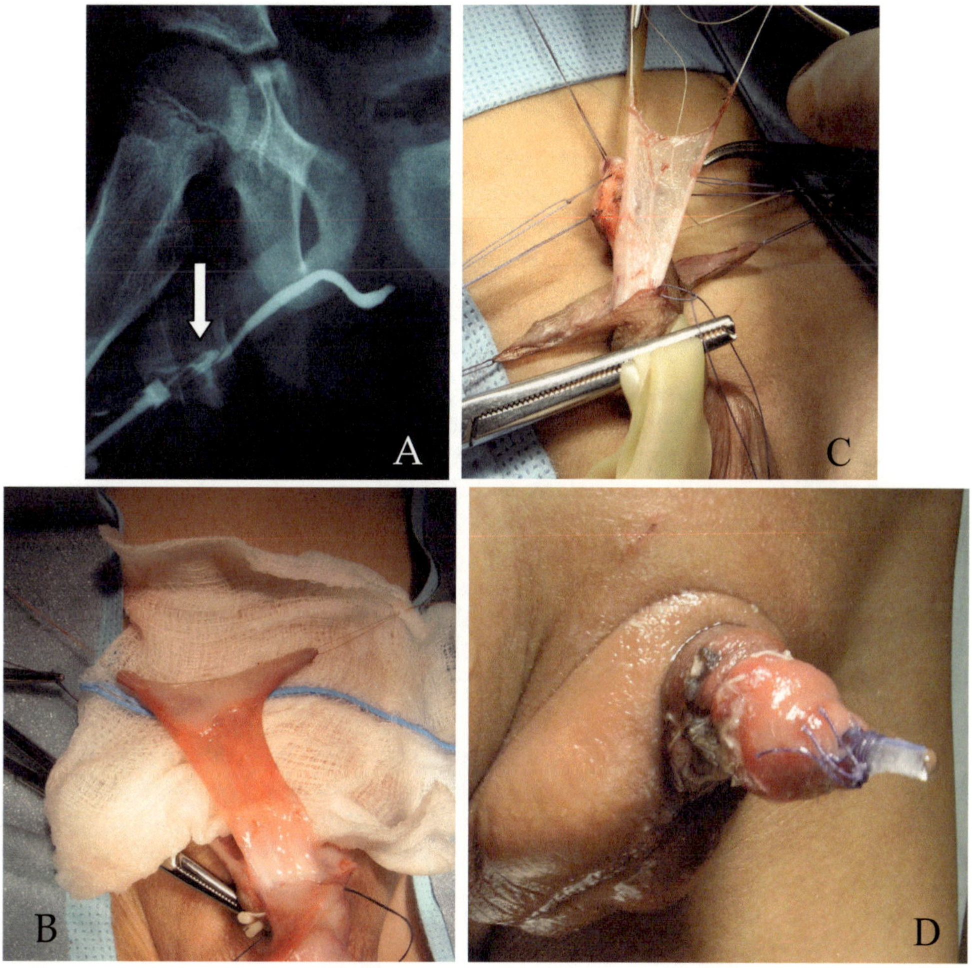

Fig. 3. Tips to minimize fistula development or recurrence: A) Preoperative contrast imaging photograph showing urethral stenosis (white arrow) and fistula after distal hypospadias repair, B) Operative photograph of the same case showing the prepared Retik's dorsal - subcutaneous preputial flap from the foreskin dorsal as a second protective layer with part of fore skin attached at tip of flap, C) Operative photograph of another case showing the dorsal dartos fascia flap prepared as a second covering layer for the urethroplasty and D) Operative photograph of a case showing the urethral stent at the time of recovery. [Courtesy of Prof. Sherif Shehata]

6.2 Protective intermediate layer

Multiple layer closure has a major role in lowering the incidence of fistula formation. The introduction of a protective intermediate layer is the most important single factor in reducing the incidence of fistula and other complications of hypospadias repair. One or more layers was essential as a protective intermediate layer between the neo urethra and the skin layer.

Types of protective intermediate layer including the following as summarized below:

- Buck`s fascia,
- Smith's de-epithelialised skin,
- Snow's tunica vaginalis wrap from the testicular coverings,
- Retik's dorsal - subcutaneous preputial flap from the foreskin,
- Motiwala's dartos flap from the scrotum
- Dorsal dartos fascia flap, and
- The external spermatic fascia flap [16, 30].

Nowadays the use of spongioplasty is important to be added as an intermediate layer and is helpful to protect the urethroplasty. Another point is the two layers closure of the glans as additional support as proved statistically in hypospadias surgery whether primary or complicated case [33].

6.3 Urethral stenting

In a prospective comparative study in Cairo University, the role of stenting and catheterization has been evaluated. The study included 100 patients divided randomly into a silicone stent group and a no stenting group. Although the difference was not statistically significant, the incidence of complications and fistula formation was higher in the stented group [13, 16]. However, if the surgeon prefers to use catheters or stents, non-reactive silicone stents or catheters are better employed. A stent or catheter one size smaller than the urethra should be selected to permit voiding around the tube should it become plugged or should bladder spasms occur. Urethral stent is superior to catheterization in post operative period regarding the surgical outcome [13, 33, 34].

6.4 Dressing

Another major factor is the use of different types of dressings. In a comparative prospective study in Cairo University, the role of dressing has been evaluated. The study concluded that dressings in general statistically increase the incidence of complications and fistula formation in hypospadias repair [14, 33]. Our experiences with others advocate the non wetting or even dryness of wound by no dressing [13, 14, 22]. Other authors showed that dressings should be omitted from routine use after hypospadias repair [13, 14, 22, 40]. For those surgeons who still prefer to use dressings, modern hypospadias dressings with materials such as Duoderm or silicone foam have also aided in reducing the incidence of fistula [15].

6.5 Tisseel

A fibrin glue preparation is used to augment hypospadias repairs in children. When this adjunct was used, the fistula rate was lowered to 9% versus 28% as reported [28, 29]. Use of fibrin sealant reduces the overall complication rate in hypospadias repair [1, 22]. Recently, the use of butyl cyanoacrylate tissue glue for post hypospadias repair dressing is of many advantages including dry sealant, transparent and protective water proof as a coated film cheaper sealant dressing from our current experience [1, Shehata, submitted].

7. Management of fistula

Every case of fistula especially if recurrent should be investigated thoroughly prior to surgery either to define possible associated anomalies or causes of recurrence such as presence of a urethral diverticulum or distal urethral stricture, as it may lead to recurrence of the fistula. The distal urethra must be examined for evidence of obstruction by cystoscopy, retrograde urethrography, ascending urethrography or urethral calibration. Intra operative calibration is of paramount importance especially with failure of tube passage. Meticulous penile examination is mandatory to assess the status of local tissue and design the management plan. Any obstruction found has to be corrected simultaneously with the fistula repair [8, 15].

Timing of the repair of post hypospadias fistula remains one of the most important issues in the outcome of repair. Once a fistula has formed, there may be inflammation and urine extravasation and urethral tissues quickly become edematous and friable. There is little point in attempting to close a newly formed fistula by means of secondary sutures, and in fact further inflammation will result in a larger fistulous opening [15, 26]. Once a fistula has formed, it is recommended that no surgical repair be considered for 6-12 months. Evermore, should all remnants of suture materials disappeared before any attempt for repair. This is the minimum time required for complete wound healing and to allow for full resolution of scar tissue. When we encountered with a recurrent fistula, the waiting time should be a minimum of one year lapse from the former repair. In some recurrent or mega fistulae the two – stage repair is advocated [35].

The classic management consist of small fistula which may heal spontaneously within 10 - 21 days of urinary diversion, with appropriate antibiotics until tissue induration and inflammation disappears when there is no meatal stenosis. Spontaneous closure of fistula has been reported in up to 30% cases. During this time, meatus can be dilated with an ophthalmic ointment tube tip to ensure an adequate meatal caliber. Dilation protocol is helpful in pin point cases of fistula provided that there is no distal or meatal stenosis [17, 20]. However, some hypospadias surgeons deny the importance of catheter as it is possible that fistulas which heal in this way would have healed in any case, without a catheter which may cause irritation that diminishes the chances of spontaneous healing [17, 28].

8. Surgical treatment

As common in hypospadias surgery, there are no perfect surgical techniques for repairing urethrocutaneous fistulae. Many variable factors could influence the surgical management and outcome of urethrocutaneous fistula repair as the time of occurrence after urethroplasty, the location (glanular, coronal, mid-shaft, etc.), size (pin-point, large), the number and the condition of local tissue [26].

During the last decade many principles of an ideal repair of fistulae have been clarified. We use the same principles that apply exactly to hypospadias repair in fistula closure and/or repair. Delicate tissue handling, delicate instruments, healthy tissue should be incorporated, a multilayer repair with well-vascularized tissues, avoiding overlapping sutures and non absorbable or thick suture materials, a tension-free closure, use of optical magnification and needle-point cautrey or bipolar cautery for coagulation are currently considered mandatory [28]. A pivotal factor is the operating surgeon that should have a fast experience in the field of hypospadiology not the surgeon who operate occasionally such cases [Warren Snodgrass, Personal Communication].

Before attempting any surgical repair of a fistula, it is important to identify the presence of a urethral diverticulum or distal urethral stricture, so the intra operative calibration of the distal urethra and distension of the repaired hypospadias to search for a diverticulum with meticulous penile examination is mandatory to assess the status of local tissues and design the management plan. Any obstruction found has to be corrected simultaneously with the fistula repair [28].

The next step is to identify the location of the fistula and to exclude any further fistulas by retrograde injection of a diluted povidone-iodine solution or methylene blue dye in to the meatus while the bulbous urethra is being compressed to prevent instillation into the bladder [13, 28].

Generally, the repair of post hypospadias fistulae depends on the size and location of the fistula. However there are many golden principles of the fistula repair which must be followed as the debridement, dissection of the fistula; elaborate excision of the fistulous tract – including the fistula cornu- down to healthy thin urethral tissue, closing by inverting suture, and protective layer closure with lastly coverage using small skin flap [8].

Many techniques advocated included; the trap door technique, simple closure, envelop like closure, using of any of the hypospadias repair techniques like TIP principle or Koff's urethral mobilization in special indications. No single technique is ideal, so the hypospadiologist should tailor the technique according to each case individually. The main two bases are tension free urethral closure and multi layer closure for protection. Also, the former technique employed in hypospadias repair is important with the status of the urethral plate to build up our technique of repair accordingly [34].

Some surgeons advised the use of purse string sutures as a simple method to close fistula which may be of value in small sized fistulae only. Although this principle carries the risk of tension at the edge of the fistula opening also its interrupted sutures; in spite of its simplicity it also had the possibility of impeded urethral epithelium in between the sutures [10].

For a small fistula, simple transverse approximation of healthy urethral tissue is often possible. Subcuticular continuous sutures of 7-0 Vicryl are used to close the urethral edges and had the benefits for preventing the leakage of the urine and passing the urethral epithelium through the sutures. Some surgeons prefer to irrigate the urethra with proximal compression intra operatively to ensure water - tight closure although it is not really necessary [19].

A protective intermediate layer plays an important part in avoiding recurrence as described before since many types of protective intermediate layer are available including; Buck's fascia, Smith's de-epithelialized skin, Snow's tunica vaginalis wrap from the testicular coverings, Retik's dorsal - subcutaneous flap from the foreskin, Motiwala's dartos flap from the scrotum, and the external spermatic fascia flap [16]. Even, the use of urethral mobilization without any suture line for distal fistulae is advocated to resolve the problem of distal fistula [17, 20, 28].

Many of the techniques used in primary repair of hypospadias are exactly used in the repair of post hypospadias urethral fistula especially if multiple or mega fistulae. In the large fistulae, the temptation to simply close the fistula is dangerous, as recurrent fistulae are quite common. Mega fistula should be managed as disrupted case of repair. Often it is advisable to repeat the whole urethroplasty [7, 34, 35].

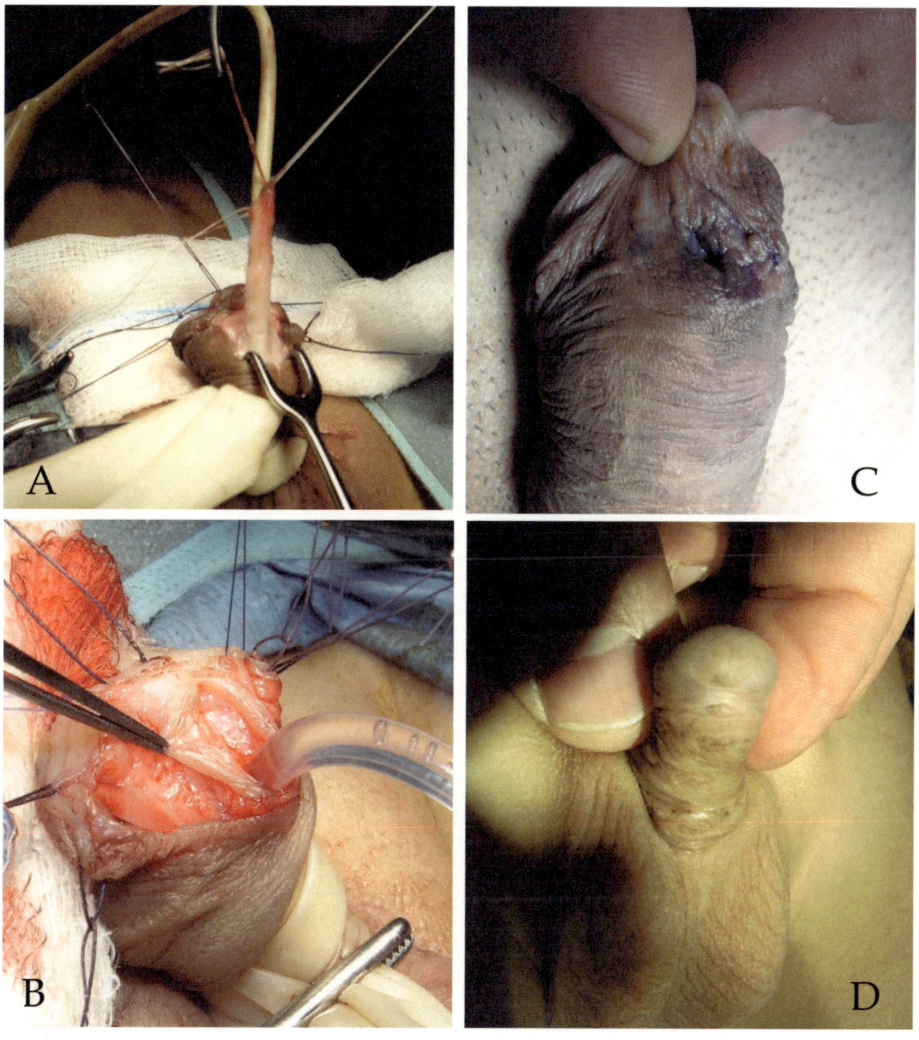

Fig. 4. Identification and techniques of fistula repair: A) Operative photograph of a case of coronal fistula treated by Koff's urethral mobilization, B) Operative photograph of a coronal fistula case converted into coronal type of hypospadias and repaired by TIP procedure, C) Preoperative photo of a coronal mega fistula with methylene blue come out of the fistula, and D) Post operative photo of small coronal fistula with skin bridge. [Courtesy of Prof. Sherif Shehata]

Most surgeons preferred converting large coronal fistulae developed after hypospadias repair, followed by tabularization of the urethral plate with or without a dorsal midline relaxing incision [2, 26, 35]. The Thiersch tube repair with or without the relaxing urethral plate incision, as described by Reddy [25], Rich et al [27] and Snodgrass [38] had a success rate of 92%. Secrest et al [31], reported on the successful urethrocutaneous fistula repair in 53 (91.4%) of the total 58 patients after hypospadias repair with converting the fistula in the primary hypospadias repair. We recently reported success rate of mega fistula by TIP principle of nearly 90 % [35].

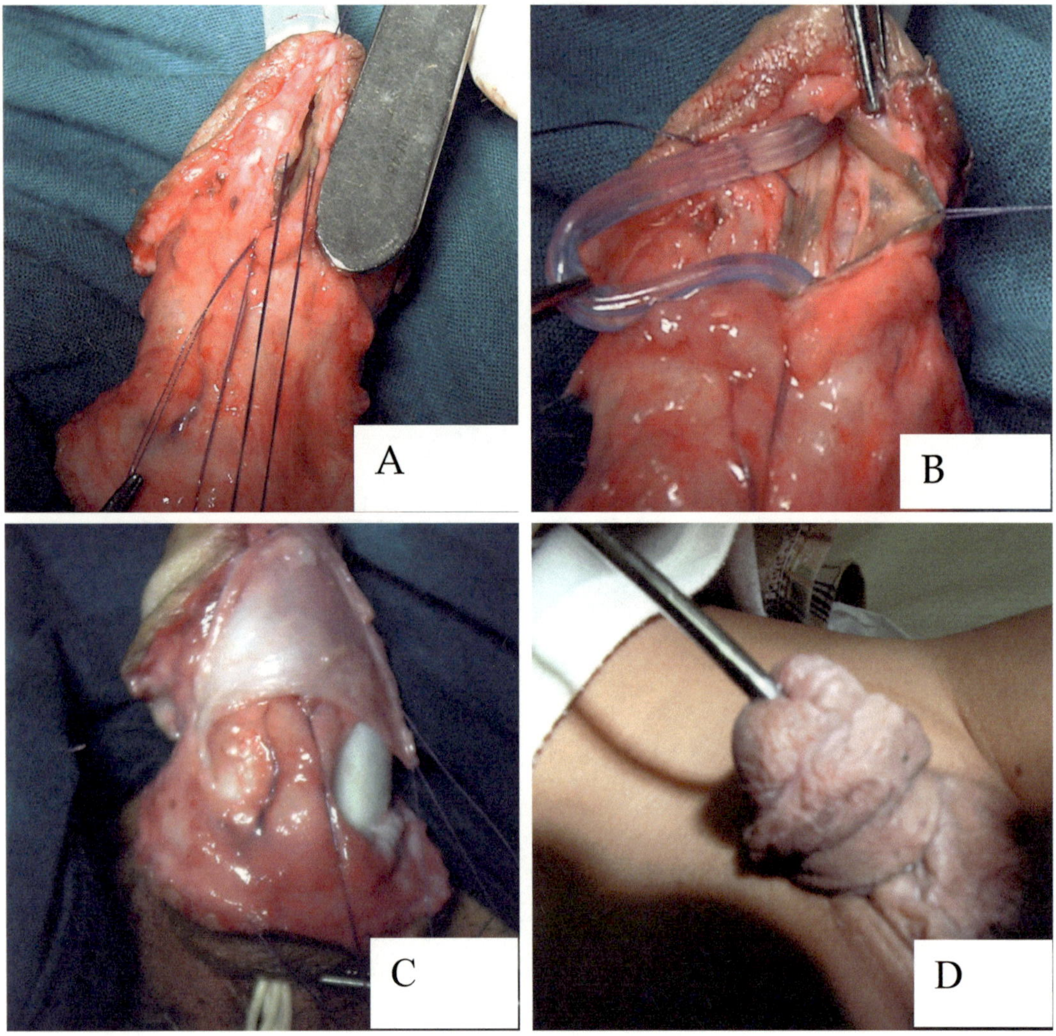

Fig. 5. Mega fistula repair by TIP principle: A) Operative photograph of penile mega fistula as compared to scalpel hand, B) Operative photograph of the same case after excision of fistula cornu and edge of healthy tissue with dorsal slit employing TIP principle, C) Operative photograph of the same case after fashioning lateral Buck's fascia protective layer and D) Post operative photograph of the same case after 3 months at calibration with complete healing. [Courtesy of Prof. Sherif Shehata]

A fistula near the glans with thin skin distally can be repaired by connecting the skin between the meatus and the fistula. The defect then is closed using the Mathieu technique to cover over the new subglanular meatus. In this technique, either a ventral or an oblique or lateral strip of skin can be used to cover over the meatus as in the classic Mathieu procedure [32].

Sometimes, the fistulous tract goes a long way before opening into the skin and there may be multiple tiny tracts that are not seen except during dissection. So it is very important to dissect and separate widely between the urethra and the overlying. Among these

techniques, the most common maneuver is to place some intervening layer of tissue between neo-urethra and the skin [4]. For multiple fistulae, a single-stage procedure is still a valid option. Two-stage procedures may be reserved for recurrent fistula where there is a deficiency of adequate healthy local tissue. In cases of serpentine, tortuous or long fistulae, it is advisable to make endoscopic treatment either by laser coagulation and fibrin glue as dissection between layers can destroy the original repair in cases of minute fistulae [16, 31].
Suture tracks (or sinuses) occur when epithelium grows along skin sutures before they dissolve or are removed postoperatively. These sinuses subsequently fill with desquamated keratin, producing unsightly marks. The likelihood that wound closure will leave suture tracks depends upon a variety of factors, including the size and composition of suture materials [39].
Recently, some surgeons have recommended the use of cyanoacrylate for repair of early fistula after hypospadias surgery and found effective. However the results are lacking the evidence yet. Endoscopic procedures even tried in some occasions [20].
Fistulae may recur because of technical errors. Contributing factors include inadequate layers of closure, ischemic tissue, and overlapping suture lines. Infection, tension such as is created by edema or hemorrhage, pressure of dressings and occlusion of catheters with urinary extravasation all contribute to fistula recurrence that should be prevented and revised step by step during repair [28]. Hence despite that some literature reports did not advocate the use of stents, our experience collected over 25 years in hypospadias field recommend the use of urethral stents for a minimum of 48 hours in distal cases following repair and suprapubic vesicostomy diversion in proximal cases.

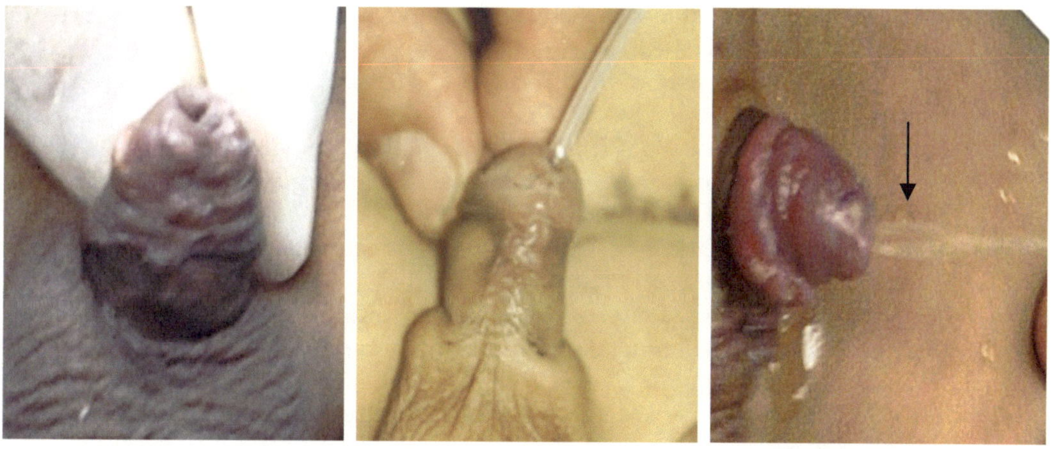

(a) (b) (c)

Fig. 6. Post operative results of fistula repair: A) Post operative photograph of a case after successful coronal fistula closure, B) Post operative photograph of another case after successful fistula closure at time of calibration, and C) Photograph of a third case at 3rd month post operative visit showing urine voiding in vertical stream (notice the black arrow) at tip of conical glans indicating the excellent result. [Courtesy of Prof. Sherif Shehata]

In conclusion, post hypospadias fistula repair need understanding of the theoretical basis and natural history of its development, technical expertise and considering the preventive measures prior to its actual development plus the honest clarification of the condition to parents and patient to participate actively in the management plan are crucial to optimize the outcome and quality of life of the affected patients.

9. References

[1] Ambriz-González, G., Velázquez-Ramírez, GA., García-González, JL., de León-Gómez, JM., Muciño-Hernández, MI., & González-Ojeda, A (2007). Use of fibrin sealant in hypospadias surgical repair reduces the frequency of postoperative complications. *Urol Int*, 78, 37- 41

[2] Awad, MS (2006). Urethral advancement technique for repair of distal penile hypospadias: A revisit. *Indian J Plast Surg*, 39, 34-38

[3] Barbagli, G., Palminteri, E., & Lazzeri, M (2001). Long-term outcome of urethroplasty after failed urethrotomy versus primary repair. *J Urol*, 165, 1918-1919

[4] Djordjevic, ML., Perovic, SV., & Vukadinovic, VM (2005). Dorsal dartos flap for preventing fistula in the Snodgrass hypospadias repair. *BJU Int*, 95, 1303-1309

[5] Dodson, L., Baird, D., Baker, L., Docimo, S., & Mathews, I (2007). Outcomes of delayed hypospadias repair: Implications for decision making. *Urology*, 11, 178, 278–281

[6] Dubois, R., Pelizzo, G., Nasser, H., Valmalle, A., & Dodat, H (1998). Urethral fistulas after surgical treatment of hypospadias: A propose of a series of 74 cases. *Prog Uro*, 8, 1029-1034

[7] Edney, MT., Lopes, JF., Schned, A., Ellsworth, PI., & Cendron, M (2004). Time course and histology of urethrocutaneous fistula formation in a porcine model of urethral healing. *Eur Urol*, 45, 806–810

[8] ElBakry, A (2001). Management of urethrocutaneous fistula after hypospadias repair: 10 years' experience. *B J U Int*, 88, 590-595

[9] El-Mahrouky, A., McElhaney, 1., & Bartone, FF (1987). In vitro comparison of the properties of polydioxanone, polyglycolic acid and catgut sutures in sterile and infected urine. *J Uro*, 138, 913-915

[10] Fatah, MF (1982). A method of closing urethral fistulae using a purse-string or interrupted silk sutures. *Br J Plast Surg*, 35, 102-103

[11] Gardikis, S., Solutanidis, C., Deftereos, S., Kambouri, K., Limas, C., & Vaos, G (2004). Suprapubic catheter knotting: An unusual complication. *Int Urol Nephrol*, 36, 537–539

[12] Greenfield, SP., Sadler, PT., & Wan, J (1994). Two stage repair for severe hypospadias. *J Uro*, 152, 498-501

[13] Hadidi, A., Abdaal, N., & Kaddah, S (2003). Hypospadias repair: is stenting important? *Kasr El Ainy J Surg*, 4. 2, 3-8

[14] Hadidi, A., Abdaal, N., & Kaddah, S (2003). Hypospadias repair: is dressing important? *Kasr El Ainy J Surg*, 4.1, 37-44.

[15] Hadidi, AT (2004). Complications and Late Sequelae, in: *Hypospadias Surgery An Illustrated Guide.* Ahmed T. Hadidi and Amir F.Azmy, 23: 273-283, Springer-Verlag, Berlin Heidelberg, New York

[16] Hadidi, AT., & Azmy, AF (2004). Editorial Overview of the Current Management of Hypospadias, In: *Hypospadias Surgery An Illustrated Guide.* Ahmed T. Hadidi and Amir F. Azmy, 35: 339-341, Springer-Verlag, Berlin, Heidelberg, New York

[17] Hayashi, Y., Mogami, M., & Kojima, Y (1998). Results of closure of urethrocutaneous fistulas after hypospadias repair. *Int J Urol*,5, 167–169

[18] Horton, C E., & Devine, C J. (1973). Urethral fistula, In: *Plastic and reconstructive surgery of the genital area.* Horton CE, 397- 403, Little & Brown Co, 12567, Boston

[19] Khan, U., Zic, R., & Boorman, J (2001). Water-proofing in hypospadias: A refinement of the two-stage reconstruction. *Br J Plast Surg*,54, 528-531

[20] LaPointe, SP., N-Fékété, C., & Lortat-Jacob, S (2002). Early closure of fistula after hypospadias surgery using N-butyl cyanoacrylate: Preliminary results. *J Urol*,168, 1751–1753

[21] Latifoglu, O., Yavuzer, R., Unal, S., Cavuonlu, T., & Atabay, K (2000). Surgical treatment of urethral fistulas following hypospadias repair. *Ann Plast Surg*,7, 44, 381- 386

[22] McLorie, G., Joyner, B., & Herz, D (2001). A prospective randomized clinical trial to evaluate methods of postoperative care of hypospadias. *J Urol*, 2, 165, 1669- 1672

[23] Mouriquand, PD., & Mure, PY(2004). Current concepts in hypospadiology. *B J U Int*, 93, 26, 120 -131

[24] Ratan, SK., Sen, A., Pandey, RM., Hans, C., Roychaudhary, S., & Ratan J (2001). Lesser evaluated determinants of fistula formation in children with hypospadias. *Int J Clin Pract* ,55, 96–99

[25] Reddy, LN (1975). One-stage repair of hypospadias. *Urology*,5, 475-478

[26] Retik, AB., Keating, M., & Mandell, J (1988). Complications of hypospadias repair. *Urol Clin North Am*,15, 223-236

[27] Rich, MA., Keating, MA., Snyder, HM., & Duckett, JW (1989). Hinging the urethral plate in hypospadias meatoplasty. *J Urol*,142, 1551-1553

[28] Richter, F., Pinto, PA., Stock, JA., & Hanna, MK (2003). Management of recurrent urethral fistulas after hypospadias repair. *Urology*, 61, 448-451

[29] Rickwood, A., & Fearne, C (1997). Pedicled penile skin for hypospadias 'rescue'. *Br J Urol*, 8, 80, 145-146

[30] Saleh M., Mohamed, N., Esmael, T., & Khaled, S (2010). A simple procedure for management of urethrocutaneous fistulas: post-hypospadias repair. *Afr J Paediatr Surg*,7, 124-128

[31] Secrest CL, Jordan GH, Winslow BH, Horton CE, McCraw JB, & Gilbert DA (1993). Repair of the complications of hypospadias surgery. *J Urol*, 150: 1415-1418

[32] Shapiro, SR (1984). Complications of hypospadias repair. *J Uro*, 11, 131, 5-18

[33] Shehata, SMK, El-Heindey MH, & El-Bahnasy AM (2006). Glanular closure during the tubularized incised plate procedure: A prospective randomized study. *Ann Pediatr Surg*, 2, 1, 39-44

[34] Shehata, SMK, Elian AA, Soliman SM, & Hassan HS (2007). Re-Operative mid penile hypospadias repair: Experience in 34 cases. *Ann Pediatr Surg*, 3, 3, 156-163

[35] Shehata, SMK (2009). Use of TIP principle for the repair of non-glanular recurrent post hypospadias urethrocutaneous mega fistula. *Eur J Ped Surg*, 19 (6), 395-398

[36] Smith, ED (1990). Hypospadias, In: *Ashcraft Pediatric Urology.* Ashcraft K, 353-395, Saunders, Philadelphia.

[37] Smith, ED (1981). Durham Smith repair of hypospadias. *Urol Clin North Am*, 8, 451-455
[38] Snodgrass, W (1994). Tubularized incised plate urethroplasty for distal hypospadias. *J Urol*, 151, 464-465
[39] Snodgrass W (1999). Suture tracts after hypospadias surgery. *BJU Int.* 84: 843-847
[40] Van Savage, JG., Palanca, LG., & Slaughenhoupt, BL (2000). A prospective randomized trial of dressings versus no dressings for hypospadias repair. *J Urol*, 164, 981- 983

6

The Treatment of Panurethral Strictures

Yue-Min Xu and Chao Feng
Department of Urology, Sixth People's Hospital, Urethral Reconstruction Center, Jiaotong University of Shanghai, Shanghai 200233, China

1. Introduction

Extensive or panurethral strictures that involve both the pendulous and bulbar urethra were difficult to treat surgically. Successful repair of panurethral strictures was challenging, particularly in patients with recurrent panurethral strictures after previous surgical attempts. Such therapeutic efforts were well-known risk factors for the failure of urethroplasty, because of spongiofibrosis and poor vascular supply. Such strictures were traditionally managed with 2-stage repairs using scrotal skin (1, 2). However, as the field of urethral reconstruction developed, there was a move towards 1-stage repair using free grafts made of skin, pedicle-based flaps or combined approaches (3-9). Numerous substitution urethroplasty techniques have been described and there were, however, no universally accepted graft material for either primary urethral substitution or technique of reconstruction after multiple failed attempts. (3-9).

The penile skin flap provided a versatile mechanism for achieving excellent results in the single-stage repair of complex anterior urethral strictures. The distal penile circular fasciocutaneous flap (FCF) technique of urethroplasty was first reported in 1993 by McAninch (10). The flap meets all criteria for tissue transfer and urethral reconstruction. It reliably provides ample hairless tissue, usually 13 to 15 cm long (depending on penile size), flexibility, versatility, and without compromising cosmesis or function (11). In addition, the circular fasciocutaneous penile flap is easily combined with other tissue-transfer techniques when necessary, enabling one-stage reconstruction in the majority of cases.

For those patients in whom genital skin was insufficient or panurethral strictures involving more than the distal bulbar urethra, alternative tissue or combined grafts urethroplasty was needed for urethral reconstruction. Wessells et al (3) reported a series of seven patients with pan-urethral strictures (mean length, 19 cm.) treated using a fasciocutaneous flap combined with buccal mucosa, bladder epithelium or skin grafts. Elliott et al (4) described nine patients who underwent distal penile fasciocutaneous flap repair of a concomitant penile urethral stricture and buccal graft reconstruction for a bulbar stricture; the repair was successful in eight of the nine patients. Berglund et al (5) reported a series of 18 patients with a mean stricture length of 15.1 cm using combined buccal mucosal graft and genital skin flap for reconstruction of extensive anterior urethral strictures.

For those patients in whom no adequate donor skin was available for grafting because of multiple penile surgeries or diseased skin existing, mucosal grafts urethroplasty may be appropriate (7,8). Several experimental studies and clinical experiences have contributed to the development and evolution of substitute urethroplasty in surgical treatment of penile and bulbar urethral strictures. In 2002 and 2003, we described the results of a pilot study on the use of the colonic mucosa as a novel substitute for urethral reconstruction in 10 dogs before performing the operation in 16 patients with severe lengthy urethral stricture (7,12,13). In 2009, we reported a series of 35 patients with a mean stricture length of 15.1 cm and mean followup 53.6 months (range 26 to 94) using colonic mucosal graft for reconstruction of extensive urethral strictures (14).

This chapter will focus on combined the penile skin flap and mucosal graft urethroplasty, combined two oral mucosal grafts urethroplasty, or colonic mucosa graft urethroplasty for urethral reconstruction. We will also review the technical aspects of staged urethroplasty.

2. Preoperative evaluation

The patient's clinical history, as well as the stricture etiology, location, and length must be carefully examined to better define the characteristics needed in substitution urethroplasty. Preoperative retrograde urethrography was mandatory to evaluate the site, number, length of stricture and the urethral plate, and voiding cystourethrography was useful in evaluating continence of the bladder neck and urethral dilation proximally to the stenosis (Fig. 1a-d). Sonourethrography and urethroscopy were suggested to collect more detailed information on stricture characteristics, especial for posterior urethra (Fig. 2a,b).

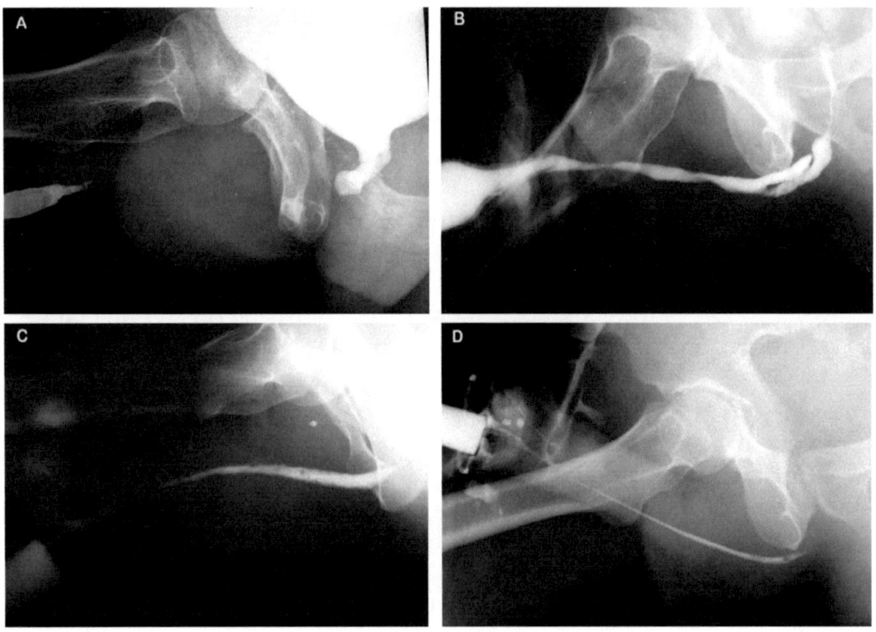

Fig. 1. Retrograde urethrography demonstrated a long segment urethral occlusion (A), multiple strictures and pseudopath (B) or long, severe stricture (C,D) in anterior urethra

Patients selected for one-stage procedure should be informed that early or later complications, such as hematoma, infection, meatal stenosis or fistula may occur with any surgical technique. The patient requiring a penile flap one-stage urethroplasty must be carefully reviewed and the genitalia meticulously inspected taking into consideration glan's shape,

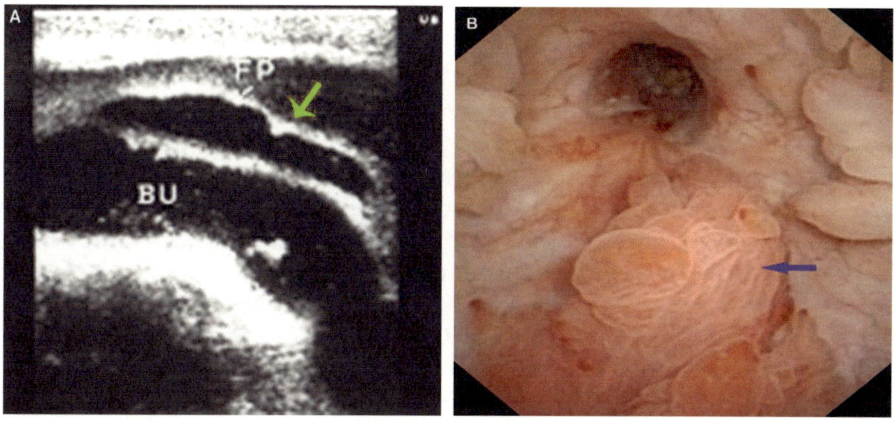

Fig. 2. (A) sonourethrogram demonstrated a pseudopath in bulbar urethra; (B) urethroscopy suggested a rigid bladder neck and neoplasm

scars in the penile and scrotal skin, the presence of residual foreskin, hair in the meatus or stones in the urethra. In addition, the presence of Lichen Sclerosus disease must be excluded (Fig. 3a-c).

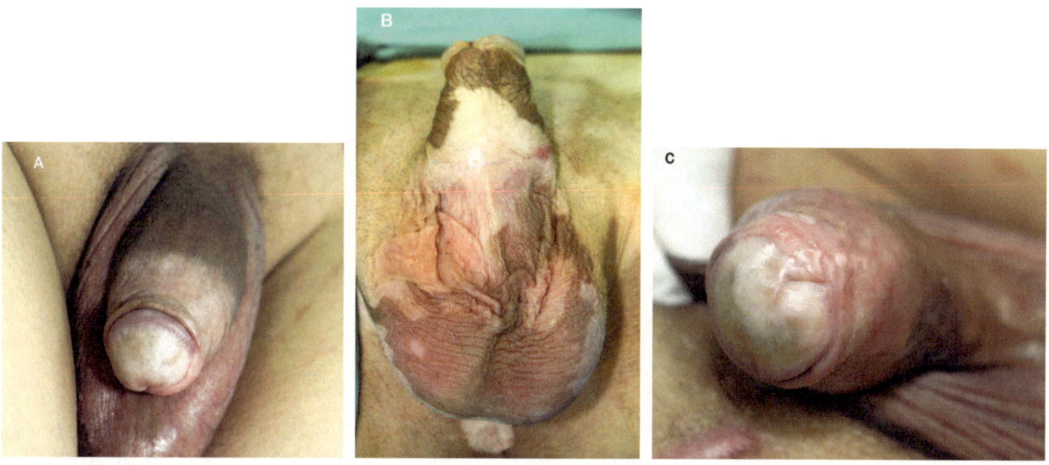

Fig. 3. LS affecting the entire glans (A), penile and scrotum skin (B), severe meatal stenosis (C)

The patient requiring an oral mucosa graft one-stage urethroplasty should be informed that oral cleansing. Two days before surgery, the patient should begin using 0.5% metronidazole mouthwash and continue three days following surgery. A broad-spectrum antibiotic is administered intravenously during the procedure and for three days afterward.

Patients who currently had an infectious disease of the mouth (such as Candida, Varicellavirus, or Herpes virus) or who have had previous surgery in the mandibular arch that prevented the mouth from being opened wide, colonic mucosa would be used for the urethroplasty.

The patient requiring a colonic mucosa graft one-stage urethroplasty should be informed that intestinal antisepsis. Three days before surgery, the patient should begin the intestinal preparation for operation, using orally nonabsorbable antibiotics administered.

3. Surgical techniques

The patient was placed in a normal lithotomy position and all surgeries were performed under general anesthesia.

3.1 Managing stenotic or obliterated urethra

A midline perineal incision and a circumcoronal foreskin or longitudinal penile incisions were required. The penile urethra and bulbar urethra were dissected from the corpora cavernosa only along the left. On the right side, the urethra remains attached to the corpora cavernosa for its full length, thus preserving its lateral vascular blood supply (Fig. 4a). The distal extent of the urethral stenosis was identified by gently inserting a 16-Fr catheter with a soft round tip until it meets resistance. The dorsal urethral surface was incised in the midline until the catheter tip and urethral lumen were exposed. The stricture tract was then incised along its entire length by a dorsal midline incision and for about 1 cm both proximally and distally into the healthy urethra (Fig. 4b). Once the entire stricture had been incised, the length and width of the remaining urethral plate was measured. Proximal and distal calibration of the urethra with a specially modified nasal speculum was critical for identifying any residual narrowing.

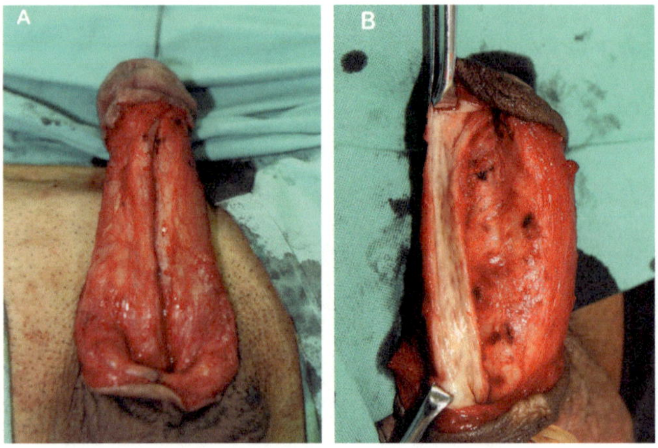

Fig. 4. (A) the penile urethra and bulbar urethra were dissected from the conpora cavernosa only along the left and remains attached to the corpora cavernosa on the right side. (B) the stricture tract was then incised along its entire length by a dorsal midline incision

For a stricture in which the lumen was more or less completely obliterated and one in which the lumen was significantly narrowed but not actually lost. For this diseased segment, we usually prefer to excise it and to replace it with mucosal grafts (Fig. 5a,b).

3.2 Oral grafts urethroplasty

Oral mucosal graft included two mucosal grafts (buccal and lingual mucosa). Since 1993 El-Kasaby et al reported the first experience with buccal mucosa urethroplasty for treatment of penile and bulbar urethral strictures (15), buccal mucosa has become an increasingly popular graft tissue for penile or bulbar urethral reconstruction performed in single or multiple stages because it was readily available in all patients and was easily harvested from the cheek or lip with a concealed donor site scar (16-20).

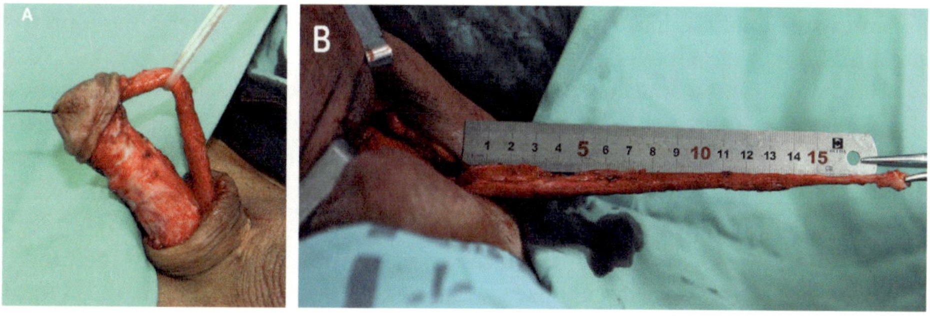

Fig. 5. (A) and (B) excising the stricture tract in which the lumen is significantly narrowed or completely obliterated

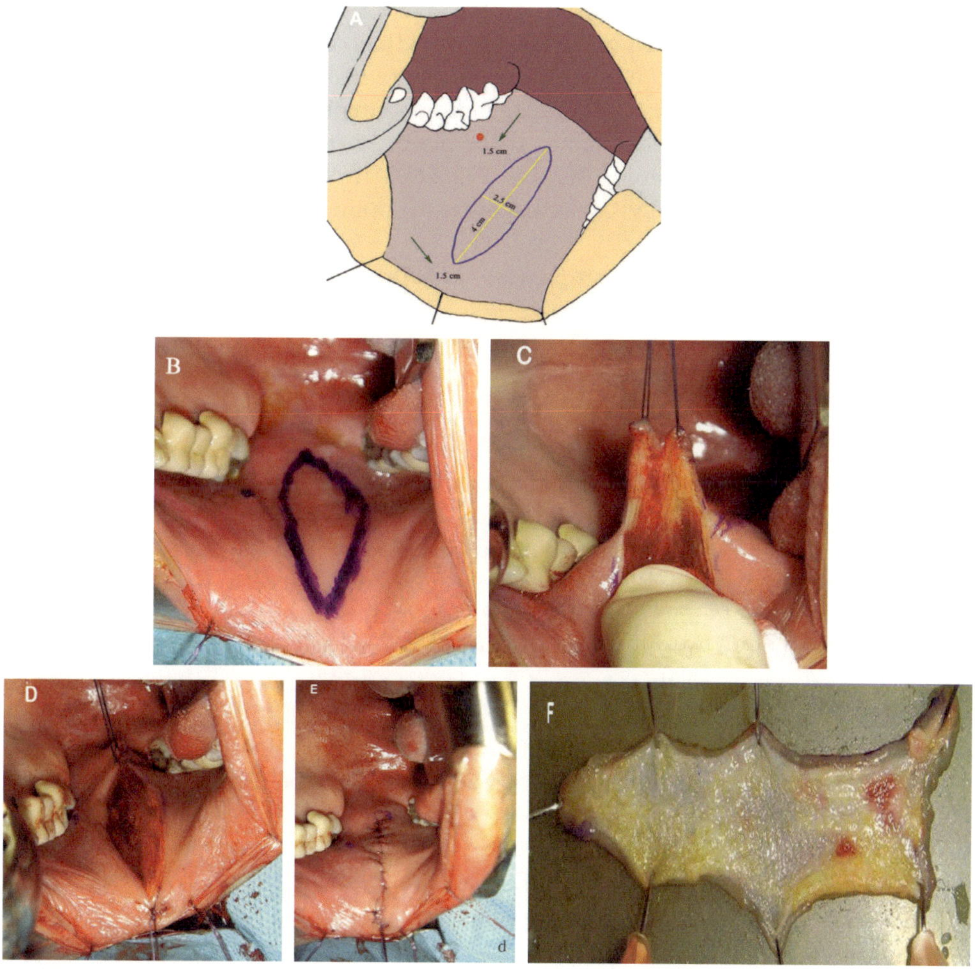

Fig. 6. The required graft marked with a surgical pen (A, B), BMG harvesting from one cheek (C), The donor site bed was carefully examined for bleeding (D) and closed using 4-0 polyglactin running sutures (E), and any excess submucosal tissue of the graft was carefully dissected away (F)

In 2006, Simonato et al first described the use of tongue tissue as an alternative donor site for graft urethroplasty and achieved good functional and aesthetic results (21,22). To further explore the use of lingual mucosa for urethral reconstruction, we investigated the use of lingual mucosa as a novel substitute for urethral reconstruction in 10 dogs before performing this operation in patients with urethral strictures (8,23,24).

3.2.1 Harvesting buccal graft

A standard mouth opener was put into place. The area to harvest was outlined and in case of buccal mucosa harvesting the Stensen's duct was identified. The required graft was measured and marked with a surgical pen (Fig. 6a,b). The area was then infiltrated with a mixed solution of 0.01‰ epinephrine plus bupivacaine to make subsequent dissection easier, minimize the amount of fat left on the undersurface of the graft and avoid dissection into the muscles (Fig. 6c). Buccal mucosal graft harvest from one cheek typically will give graft of 5cm to 6cm (depending on oral anatomy) and thus can be used to repair strictures of up to 9cm to 11cm. However, the buccal mucosa may not be useful independently for the treatment of the panurethral stricture because of limited material.

The donor site bed was carefully examined for bleeding (Fig. 6d) and the donor site was closed using 4-0 polyglactin running sutures (Fig. 6e). Any excess submucosal tissue, fat or muscle of the graft was carefully dissected away to optimize subsequent vascularization (Fig. 6f).

An ice pack was left for 6 hours postoperatively. Fluid and food intake was left up to the patient.

3.2.2 Harvesting lingual mucosal graft

A standard mouth opener was put into place. The apex of the tongue was passed through via a stitch for traction outside of the mouth to expose the ventrolateral surface of the tongue. Graft was harvested from the ventral to lateral mucosal lining of the tongue. The required graft was measured and marked with a surgical pen (Fig. 7a,b). The harvest graft site was infiltrated with a mixed solution of 0.01‰ epinephrine plus bupivacaine. The graft edges were incised and a full-thickness mucosal graft was harvested using a sharp knife beginning at the anterior landmark of the graft (Fig. 7c,d). Any excess submucosal tissue, fat or muscle of the graft was carefully dissected away to optimize subsequent vascularization. The donor site bed was carefully examined for bleeding and the donor site was closed using 4-0 polyglactin running sutures (Fig. 7e).

Bilateral lingual mucosal grafts harvested from the tongue typically will give grafts of 10 cm to 14 cm (Fig. 7f,g) (depending on tongue size), and thus can be used to repair strictures of up 9 to 13cm.

3.2.3 Combined two oral grafts (buccal or lingual) urethroplasty

Most singleness oral mucosa graft may not be insufficient in length for the treatment of the panurethral stricture and combined two oral mucosa grafts (buccal mucosa or lingual mucosa) were always required.

One or two oral mucosa grafts (buccal or lingual grafts) were trimmed to an appropriate size according to the length and width of the urethrotomy. Combined buccal mucosa graft (Fig. 8a) or longer lingual mucosal graft (9 to 14 cm, Fig. 8b) (depending on the length of urethra stricture or defection) were positioned into the urethrotomy defect. Spread-fixed to the underlying corpora cavernosa and two apices of the graft were sutured to the proximal and distal apices of the urethrotomy with interrupted stitches of 5-0 polyglactin. (Fig. 8a-c). Continuous upward traction was applied to the inverted penis while applying the penile portion of the graft to prevent chordee. A Foley 16 Fr to 18 Fr soft grooved silicone catheter was inserted. The full length of the urethra was rotated to its original position over the graft on the left side (Fig. 8d,e). At the end of the procedure, the graft was completely covered by the urethra, then by the muscles. Colles' fascia, the skin were closed with interrupted absorbable sutures (Fig. 8f). The bladder was drained through a suprapubic catheter; the urethral silicone stent was left indwelling for 14-21 days.

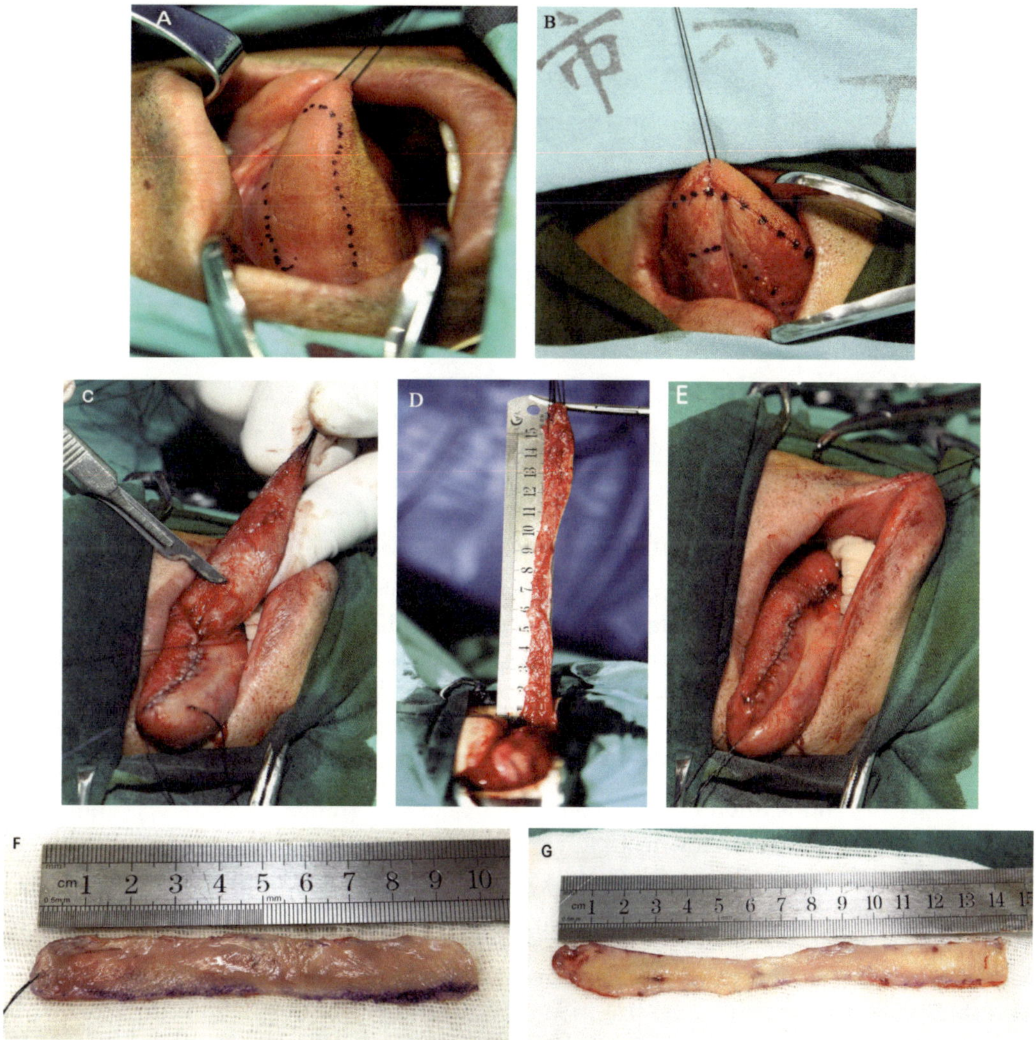

Fig. 7. The required graft marked with a surgical pen (A, B), LMG harvesting from the tongue (C) and (D), The donor site bed was closed using 4-0 polyglactin running sutures (E). Bilateral lingual mucosal grafts harvest from the tongue (F,G)

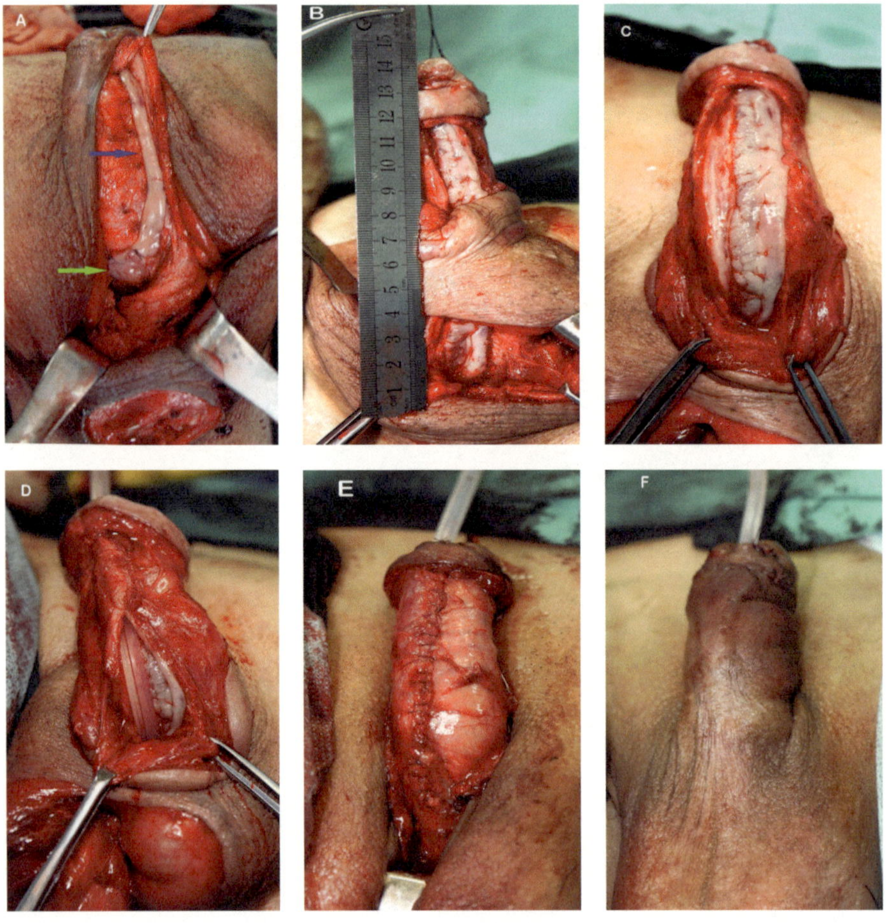

Fig. 8. Oral mucosal grafts urethroplasty. Augmentation of the urethral plate using the LMG and BMG (A), green arrow indicates LMG; blue arrow indicates BMG; LMG was positioned into the urethrotomy defect, spread-fixed to the underlying corpora cavernosa. (B), The LMG was sutured laterally to the mucosal margin of the urethral plate, augmentation of the urethral plate (C), the urethral plate sutured to mucosal margins over an 18 F soft grooved silicone catheter and the urethra was retubularized (D,E), closing the penile skin (F)

In our center, 92 consecutive patients, average age 33.8 yr (range 13 to 71 yr), underwent anterior urethra reconstruction with LMG between August 2006 and April 2009 for urethral strictures (24). Of the 92 patients, 38 patients with long-segment urethral strictures (9–18 cm) underwent dual LMG or LMG combined with foreskin flap or buccal mucosal graft urethroplasty. 34 of 38 patients were successful (89.47%) and 4 (10.53%) were failures, including urinary fistulas in one patient, recurrent stricture developed in 3 patients. We harvested grafts from both the ventral to lateral mucosa of the tongue in order to obtain a wider graft and create stable neourethras, thereby reducing the risk of recurrence at the distal or proximal graft anastomotic sites. The surgical techniques for harvesting single and double mucosal grafts from the tongue are simple and safe; and complications are rare. The tongue is an excellent source of graft material for anterior mucosal strictures. Dual LMG or combined lingual mucosa/buccal mucosa grafts and/or foreskin flap substitution urethroplasty can successfully treat longer, more complex urethral strictures.

3.3 Colonic mucosa urethroplasty

Another graft material for reconstructing the panurethral stricture was the colonic mucosa. Under general anesthesia, stricture or atretic urethra and scar tissue were excised and the penis was straightened. The length of urethra defect was measured.

3.3.1 Harvesting colonic graft

Sigmoid colon resections may be performed using laparoscopic techniques or by lower abdomen paramedian incisions, 12 to 15 cm long sigmoid colon with its blood pedicle was isolated from the intestinal tract; the digestive connection was immediately restored by an end-to-end anastomosis. Full-thickness colonic mucosal graft (15 to 22 cm in length) was harvested from the isolated colon and the isolated colon was resected afterward. After tailoring the mucosa graft, any excess submucosal tissue, fat or muscle was carefully dissected away to optimize subsequent vascularization.

3.3.2 Urethral reconstruction

An unstretched colonic mucosa was trimmed to an appropriate size according to the length (15 to 22 cm in length and 3.0 cm in width), and was tubularized over an 16 to 18 Fr fenestrated or fluted silicone tube with interrupted 5-zero polyglactin sutures to create the neourethra (Fig. 9a). End-to-end anastomosis was performed between the native urethra and the neourethra with interrupted 5-zero polyglactin sutures or one end of neourethra was anastomosed to the proximal native urethra and the other end was pulled through the glanular tunnel to form the new meatus (Fig. 9b,c). The penile skin was closed and penis was wrapped with soft, elastic, and roller bandage incorporating the traction suture into the dressing. Strips of elastic adhesive were placed over this to keep the penis in the erect position. The dressing and bolster were taken down after 3 to 5 d. The bladder was drained through a suprapubic catheter; the urethral silicone stent was left indwelling for 14-21 days.

In our center, 35 patients, average age 39.8yr (range 17 to 70yr), underwent colonic mucosal graft urethroplasty between 2000 and 2006 for complex, long-segment urethral strictures. Urethral reconstruction was performed using 11 to 21 cm (mean, 15.1) colonic mucosa grafts (14). The study demonstrates that, at a mean follow-up interval of 53.6 months, five of the 35 patients had developed recurrent strictures. However, an anastomotic site stricture developed in only one patient, and recurrent strictures in two additional patients were unrelated to the urethroplasty. Therefore, tubularized urethroplasty using colonic mucosa was associated with a lower recurrence rate than patch urethroplasty.

Colonic mucosa graft urethroplasty should be considered in patients with complex, long-segment urethral strictures. This approach may be particularly useful in patients for whom prior anterior urethroplasty was unsuccessful or in cases for where penile skin or other types of mucosal grafts are not available.

Most urethroplasty using mucosa grafts was a one-stage method for the treatment of complex urethral lengthy stricture. The key to a successful transplantation of mucosa grafts depended on whether the neovascularization was established. The following conditions were necessary for the success: 1) scar tissue should be excised as long as possible and the urethral bed for receiving the graft must be well vascularized; 2) an ischemia time of the mucosal grafts should be as short as possible; 3) to avoid wound infection and sterile urine should be ensured.

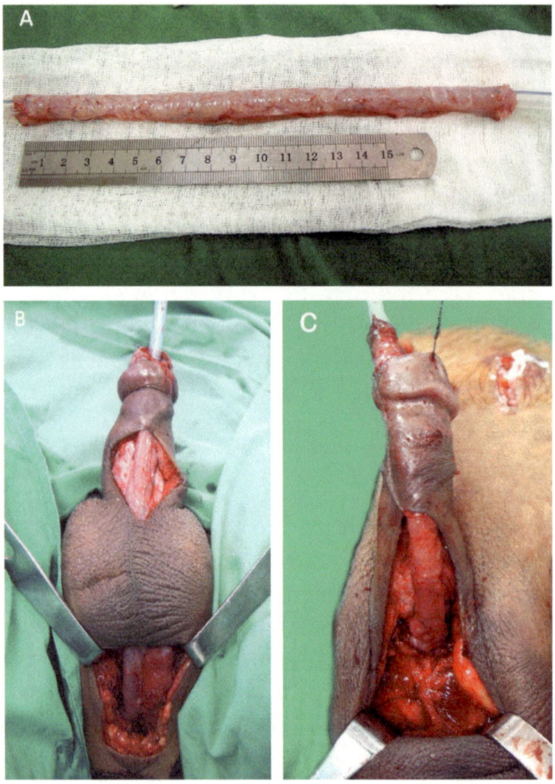

Fig. 9. A free colonic mucosa tubularized over 18 Fr silicone tube (A); colonic mucosa was anastomosed to native urethral ends (B), end of mucosa was pulled through the glanular tunnel to form the new meatus (C)

3.4 Flap combined with graft urethroplasty

For patient had a prepuce and no lichen sclerosus (LS), single-stage urethral reconstruction with a distal circumferential penile skin flap was often used to repair urethra. If the flap was insufficient or panurethral strictures involving more than the distal bulbar urethra, alternative tissue or combined grafts urethroplasty was needed for urethral reconstruction.

3.4.1 Taking penile flap

The circular pedicle island skin flap (McAninch) will typically be roughly 10~13 cm in length (depending on penile size) and 2cm in width (Fig. 10a,b). Others have used an Orandi flap in combination with a proximal graft; however, the Orandi flap was typically limited by shaft hair, and thus typically only 8-9cm in length (depending on penile size) (25).
For the distal margin of the circular skin flap, the incision was deep to the dartos of the penis and includes the anterior lamella of Buck's fascia. Such a depth was free of vascular. For the proximal margin of the skin flap, the skin was incised sharply with a scalpel, until the skin easily separates from its underlying dartos tissue. The skin can then be mobilized

away from the dartos vascular pedicle in an avascular, areolar like layer. If the pedicle of dartos and anterior lamella of Buck's fascia was adequately mobilized, the flap can be transposed even to the distal bulbar urethra, through a window underneath the scrotum.

3.4.2 Urethral reconstruction

The circular fasciocutaneous onlay flap was positioned into the urethrotomy defect and spread-fixed to the underlying corpora cavernosa. The edges of the flap were sutured to the native urethra with interrupted stitches of 5-0 polyglactin.

If the flap was insufficient in length to repair panurethral strictures, the penile urethral stricture was to repair with the flap and the bulbar stricture was to repair using an oral graft (buccal or lingual mucosa graft). The oral graft (buccal or lingual mucosa graft) was spread-fixed to the proximal bulbar urethra and the distal end of the graft was sutured to the proximal end of the flap with interrupted sutures (Fig. 10c). At the end of the procedure, the graft was completely covered by the urethra, then by the muscles. Colles' fascia, the skin were closed with interrupted absorbable sutures. The bladder was drained through a suprapubic catheter; the urethral silicone stent was left indwelling for 14-21 days.

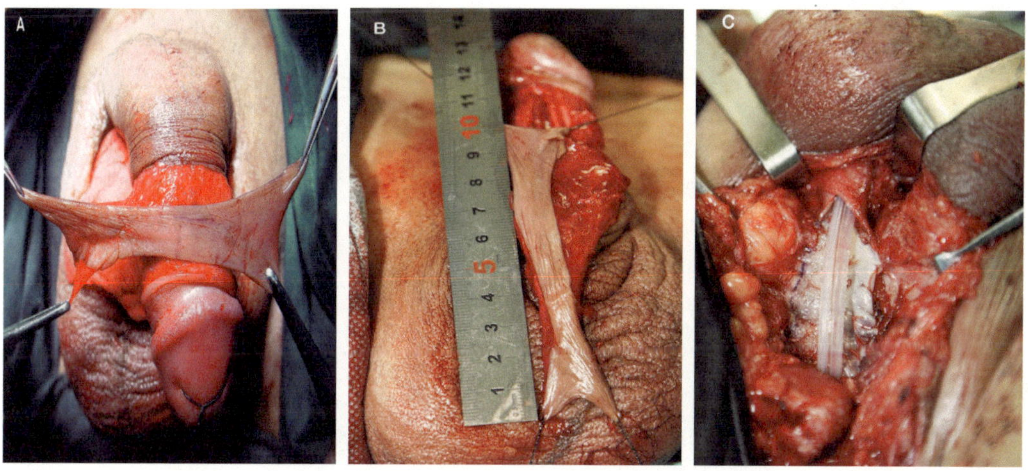

Fig. 10. A circular fasciocutaneous flap (A), fully mobilized and rotated vertically for use as an onlay flap (B). obliterated bulbar stricture was to repair using lingual mucosa graft (C)

3.5 Staged urethroplasty

For the patient with multiple surgeries and urethral infection resulting in the patient had only a 5 to 6 cm normal pendulous urethra and 2 to 3 cm prostatic urethra (Fig. 11a), the residual urethra was occlusive, and there was not enough healthy skin graft and the bed to receive the graft was not well vascularized, and where the tissues were often very scarred that had failed multiple prior urethroplasty (Fig. 11b), so substitution urethroplasty was not feasible. A staged urethroplasty may be preferable or essential (26).

3.5.1 Surgical procedures

The patient was placed in a normal lithotomy position and all surgeries were performed under general anesthesia. An inverted Y-shaped perineal incision was made, extending anteriorly to the scrotum and penis. After the scrotum was split open, the anterior urethra

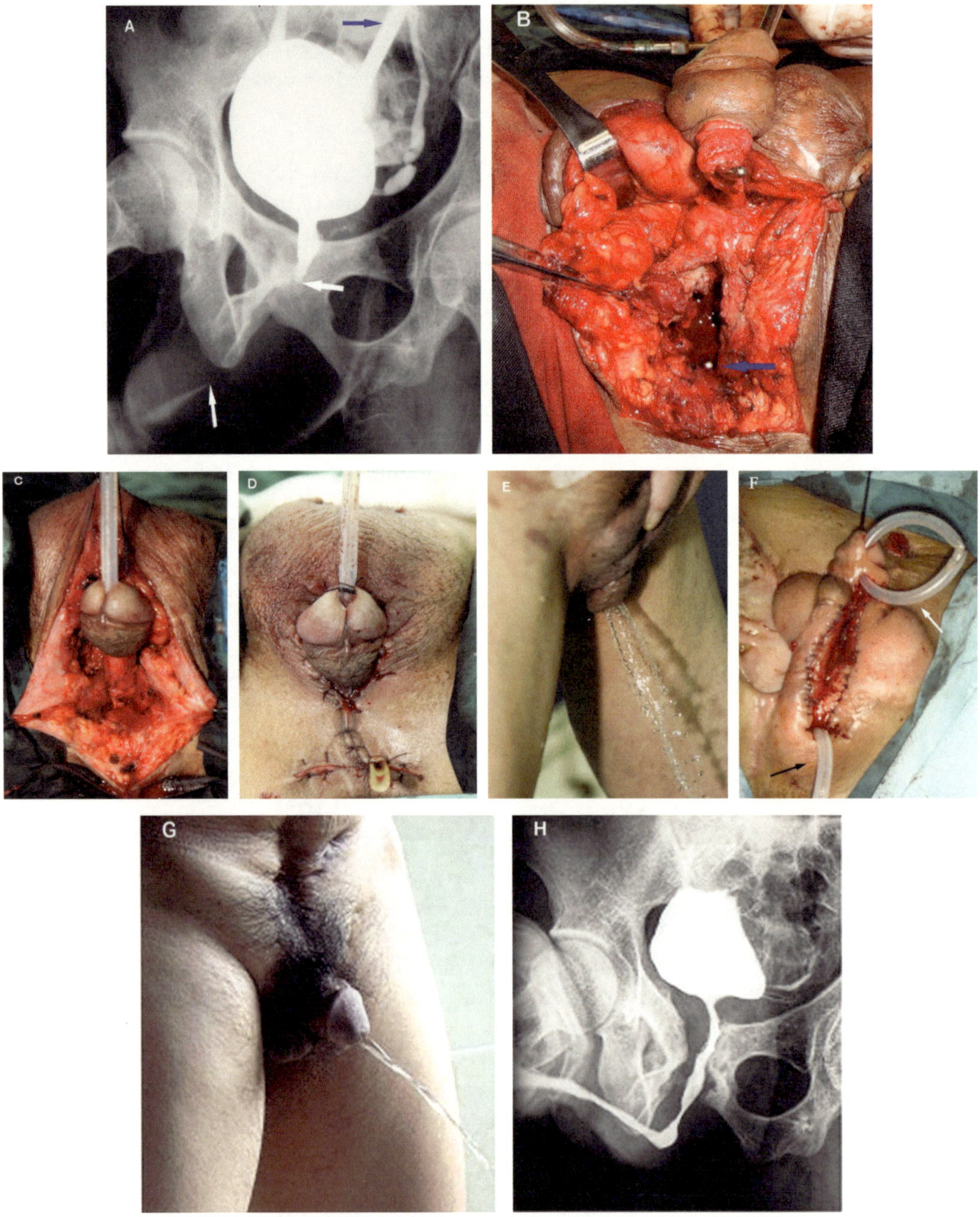

Fig. 11. (A), RUG and VUG show a shorter anterior urethra and posterior urethra, (B), transposition of penis to perineum, blue arrow indicates the distal end of posterior urethra. Pendulous-prostatic anastomostic urethroplasty (C). At the end of the procedure (D), voiding well after the first-stage op (E), straightened penis and urethroperineostomy and urethral ditch after the second-stage op (F). (G), urination after the third stage op; (H), RUG and VUG show patent urethra

was mobilized circumferentially down to the coronary sulcus (Fig. 11c). The obliterated urethra and periurethral fibrotic tissues were completely excised until a healthy prostatic urethra was mobilized about 0.5 cm for the suture. At the same time, a crural bifurcation of the corporal body separation was made. The penis and external urethral meatus were transposed to the perineum through the scrotal septum incision. The pendulous urethra was rerouted to the prostatic urethra. Tension-free pendulous-prostatic anastomotic urethroplaty was performed with the use of 4-0 polyglycolic acid sutures (Fig. 11d).
If a tension-free anastomosis could not be achieved through the perineal route; therefore, a transpubic incision and pubectomy or transperineal incision and partial inferior pubectomy should be considered. A 16 to 18 Fr fenestrated or fluted silicone tube was used as a urethral stent, a suprapubic cystostomy tube was inserted, and perineal wound was closed with a drain.
The urethral catheter was removed 21 days postoperatively. Uroflowmetry and VUG were done. If voiding was satisfactory (Fig. 11e), the suprapubic cystostomy tube was removed one day later.
The curved spongy body of the penis was separated at least 6 months later when the anterior urethra was revascularized from periurethral tissue. After the urethra was transected at the site of the coronary sulcus, the spongy body was straightened. Urethroperineostomy was performed with the proximal urethral meatus being fractionated into three valves and sutured with perineal skin. The fibrotic tissue of the albuginea penis was excised. The distal urethral stump was sutured with the skin of the penis. Skin edges of the penis and the scrotum between the urethral defects were sutured to two sides of the penile albuginea. This ventral part of the penile albuginea from the urethroperineostomy to the coronary sulcus formed an open urethral ditch that would later become epithelized. After the second-staged operation, the urethra was something like an artificial hypospadia with a normal urethral meatus (Fig. 11f).
After the urethra was transected at the site of the coronary sulcus, the spongy body was straightened, if there had a well vascularized bed to receive the graft between the proximal and distal urethral meatus, following substitution urethroplasty with oral mucosa graft between the proximal and distal urethral meatus may be preferable.
The following surgery was reconstruction of a new anterior urethra using second-stage Johanson urethroplasty. It was performed 6 months after the second surgery. A longitudinal incision of two sides of the ventral epithelized skin was made, which circled the proximal and distal meatus of the urethra, and external epithelized deep to the albuginea penis. A 1.5cm wide strip of ventral epithelized skin at the urethral ditch was used to form the dorsal wall of the new urethra. The lateral skin was undermined and closed over the buried strip to form a tube for the new urethra. In the meantime, a release incision on the dorsum of penis was made to ease the tension of the ventral wound. The ventral side of the new urethra was left to become epithelized. A suprapubic cystostomy tube was placed.
The urethral stent was removed 14 to 21 days postoperatively. If voiding was satisfactory (Fig. 11g, h), the suprapubic catheter was then removed 1 day later.

4. Selection of the urethral surgical procedures

Revisional surgery of a full-length stricture involving both the bulbar and the penile urethra was very difficult and the recurrence rate was therefore higher. Indeed the more extensive the disease, the more complicated its surgical treatment. What is the best technique to repair panurethral stricture? How to choose? There was no gold standard and was a matter of individual judgment based on experience and the circumstances. The surgical procedures for repairing a panurethral stricture in our experiences were selected according to following principle:

1. For patient had a prepuce and no lichen sclerosus (LS), single-stage urethral reconstruction with a distal circumferential skin flap has become our first choice to repair anterior urethra. If the flap was insufficient in length or panurethral strictures involving more than the proximal bulbar urethra, alternative tissue or combined oral grafts urethroplasty was needed to augment the entire bulbar urethra from the sphincter to the peno-scrotal junction (Fig. 10b,c). Most of the complications with skin flap urethroplasty were recurrent stricture, troublesome postvoid dribbing, and diverticulum formation (6).
2. Panurethral strictures were induced by lichen sclerosus (LS) and that was the complex and difficult to repair, surgery often needs to be individualized. In severe lichen sclerosus, the meatus and fossa navicularis were almost completely obliterated (Fig. 3c), wood-hard fibrosis extended into the pendulous urethra. The stenotic bands that develop were typically multiple and throughout the bulbar and pendulous urethra.

In these severe cases the penile shaft skin was often affected by LS as well (Fig. 3b) and, thus, the nonvisible, subclinical disease will often just manifest later. Therefore, the presence of lichen sclerosus has to be considered a contraindication for any type of urethroplasty involving skin. The general principle here was to excise the diseased segment and to replace it with colonic mucosal graft, because colonic mucosal graft was the material least likely to be affected by recurrent LS.

Colonic mucosa was elastic with a slight tendency to retract. Its harvesting was less difficult with good dissecting technique and the graft provided abundant material for urethroplasty. Colonic mucosal graft urethroplasty was an effective technique for the management of extensive or pan-urethral strictures. The result was good, sustained and associated with a low complication rate so that it should be performed in preference to a substitution repair when possible. Meatal or anastomosed site stenosis was seemed to have a higher risk of failure (14).

3. For patient with multiple surgeries resulting in a shortage of local skin or in medium lichen sclerosus, therefore, the urethral lumen was not significantly narrowed and the urethral plate was remaining, we usually prefer a longer lingual mucosal graft (9 to 14 cm) or combined buccal mucosa graft (depending on the length of urethra stricture or defect) to augment strictures urethra.

For meatal stricture was induced by lichen sclerosus (Fig. 12a), where the tissues were often very scarred, we favor excision of the glandular urethral plate and enlarge meatus and followed by complete replaced by mucosal grafts and a neomeatus was then made (Fig. 12b-d).

Combined dual lingual/buccal graft urethroplasty can successfully treat long urethral strictures. The surgical technique for harvesting single and double mucosal grafts from the tongue is simple, safe, and complications were rare (8).

4. If patient had only a 5 to 6 cm normal pendulous urethra and 2 to 3 cm prostatic urethra, the residual urethra was occlusive, and there was not enough healthy skin graft and the bed for receiving the graft was not well vascularized, we usually prefer a staged urethroplasty (26).

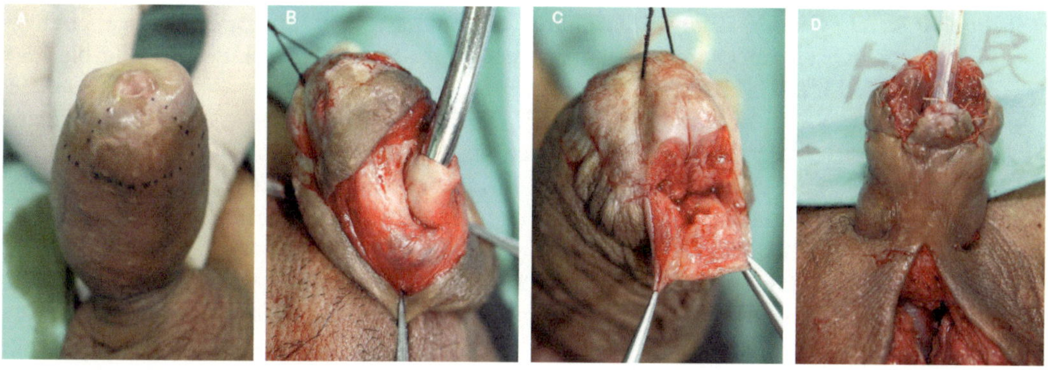

Fig. 12. Glandular reconstruction. Meatus and subcoronal incision (A), urethral plate was dissected from the glans-wings (B), excised urethral plate (C) and replaced by colonic mucosal graft (D)

5. References

[1] Johansen B. Reconstruction of the male urethra in strictures. Acta Chir Scand 1953; 176 (Suppl):1-103.

[2] Al-Ali M, Al-Hajaj R. Johanson's staged urethroplasty revisited in the salvage treatment of 68 complex urethral stricture patients: presentation of total urethroplasty. Eur Urol, 2001;39:268-71.

[3] Wessells H, Morey AF, McAninch JW. Single stage reconstruction of complex anterior urethral strictures: combined tissue transfer techniques. J Urol, 1997;157: 1271-1274.

[4] Elliott SP, Metro MJ, McAninch JW. Long-term followup of the ventrally placed buccal mucosa onlay graft in bulbar urethral reconstruction. J Urol, 2003;169:1754-1757.

[5] Berglund RK, Angermeier KW. Combined buccal mucosa graft and genital skin flap for reconstruction of extensive anterior urethral strictures. Urology, 2006; 68:707-710.

[6] Xu Y-M, Qiao Y, Sa Y-L, Wu DL, Zhang XR, Zhang J, et al. Substitution urethroplasty of complex and long-segment urethral strictures: a rationale for procedure selection. Eur Urol, 2007; 51:1093-1099,

[7] Xu Y-M, Qiao Y, Sa YL, Wu DL, Zhang J, Zhang XR, et al. 1-stage urethral reconstruction using colonic mucosa graft for the treatment of a long complex urethral stricture. J Urol, 2004; 171:220-223,

[8] Xu YM, Sa YL, Qiang Fu, Zhang J, Si JM, Liu ZS. Oral mucosal grafts urethroplasty for the treatment of long segmented anterior urethral strictures. World J Urol, 2009; 27:565-571.

[9] Barbagli G, Palminteri E, Lazzeri M, Guazzoni G. Anterior urethral strictures. BJU Int, 2003; 92:497-505

[10] McAninch JW. Reconstruction of extensive urethral strictures circular fasciocutaneous flap. J Urol, 1993; 149:488-491.

[11] Carney KJ, McAninch JW. Penile circular fasciocutaneous flaps to reconstruct complex anterior urethral strictures. Urol Clin N Am, 2002; 29:397-409

[12] Xu YM, Qiao Y, Sa YL, Zhang, HZ, Zhang, XR, Zhang J, et al.: An experimental study of colonic mucosa graft for urethral reconstruction. Chin Med J, 2002; 115:1163-1165.

[13] Xu YM, Sa YL, Qiao Y, Zhang HZ, Zhang XR, Zhang J, et al. Histopathological changes of tree buccal mucosa and colonic mucosa grafts after translation to dog bladder. Chin Med J, 2005; 118:337-339.

[14] Xu YM, Qiao Y, Sa YL, Zhang J, Jin CR, Fu Q, et al. Urethral reconstruction using colonic mucosa graft for complex strictures. J Urol, 2009; 182:1040-1043.

[15] El-kasaby AW, Fath-Alla M, Noweir AM, El-Halaby MR, Zakaria W, El-Beialy MH. The use of buccal mucosa patch graft in the management of anterior urethral strictures. J Urol, 1993; 149:276-278.

[16] Kane CJ, Tarman GJ, Summerton DJ, Buchmann CE, Ward JF, O'Reilly KJ, et al. Multi-institutional experience with buccal mucosa onlay urethroplasty for bulbar urethral reconstruction. J Urol, 2002; 167:1314–1317.

[17] Andrich DE, Mundy AR. Substitution urethroplasty with buccal mucosal free grafts. J Urol, 2001; 165:1131–1133.

[18] Patterson JM, Chapple CR. Surgical techniques in substitution urethroplasty using buccal mucosa for the treatment of anterior urethral strictures. Eur Urol, 2008; 53:1162–1171.

[19] Markiewicz MR, Lukose MA, Margarone 3rd JE, Barbagli G, Miller KS, Chuang SK. The oral mucosa graft: a systematic review. J Urol, 2007; 178:387–394.

[20] Barbagli G, Guazzoni G, Lazzeri M. One-stage bulbar urethroplasty: retrospective analysis of the results in 375 patients. Eur Urol, 2008;53:828-833.

[21] Simonato A, Gregori A, Lissiani A, Galli S, Ottaviani F, Rossi R, et al. The tongue as an alternative donor site for graft urethroplasty: a pilot study. J Urol, 2006; 175:589-592.

[22] Simonato A, Gregori A, Ambruosi C, Venzano F, Varca V, Romagnoli A, et al. Lingual mucosa graft urethroplasty for anterior urethral reconstruction. Eur Urol, 2008; 54:79-87.

[23] Song LJ, Xu YM, Hu XY, Zhang HZ. Urethral substitution using autologous lingual mucosal grafts: an experimental study. BJU Int, 2008; 101:739-743.

[24] Xu YM, Fu Q, Sa YL, Zhang J, Jin CR, Si JM, et al. Treatment of urethral strictures using lingual mucosas urethroplasty: experience of 92 cases. Chin Med J, 2010; 123:458-462

[25] Quartey JK. One-stage penile/preputial cutaneous island flap urethroplasty for urethral stricture: a preliminary report. J Urol, 1983; 129:284–287.

[26] Wu DL, Jin SB, Zhang J, Chen Y, Jin CR, Xu YM. Staged pendulous-prostatic anastomotic urethroplasty followed by reconstruction of the anterior urethra: An effective treatment for long-segment bulbar and membranous urethral stricture. European Urology, 2007; 51:504-511.

7

Complex Posterior Urethral Stricture

Ying-Long Sa and Yue-Min Xu
Department of Urology, Sixth People's Hospital, Urethral Reconstruction Center, Jiaotong University of Shanghai, Shanghai 200233, China

1. Introduction

Majority of posterior urethral stricture results from pelvic fracture, straddle injuries, or crush injuries. The management of traumatic posterior urethral strictures remains one of the most difficult tasks in urologic practice. In developed countries, agricultural activities have reduced over time and the number of accidents with pelvic fracture due to tractors tipping over has markedly decreased. Work site accidents have also markedly decreased due to the effective prevention of these kinds of accidents, and pedestrian, bicycle, and motorcycle accidents have diminished due to the increased using of cars. But patient conditions are so different from those present in developing countries, such as Egypt, India, Nepal, and China. In those countries, agricultural activities are still quite prevalent, the prevention of accidents on the work site has not dramatically lessened, and bicycles and motorcycles are the most popularly vehicles (1). Moreover, the emergency treatment of patients with PFUDDs in developing and developed countries is quite different. In Italy, emergency treatment for PFUDD was often provided by a urologist in 92.7% of cases, while in india emergency it is done by a general surgeon in 70.1% of cases. Since the majority of those patients have been treated using incorrect maneuvers in some developing country, iatrogenic damage to the urethra may be added (2). In our country, as China is large population, vast territory and uneven development of medical standards, many iatrogenic injurys were caused by inappropriate treatment, complex posterior strictures are not uncommon. Our center received nearly 200 complex posterior urethral strictures every year from all over the country. Hence, this chapter focuses on the management of traumatic posterior urethral injuries typically sustained in association with pelvic fracture.

Complex posterior urethral strictures continue to represent a genuine challenge and they pose one of the most difficult management problems in urology, which represents 5% of all urethral strictures. It is characterized by a stricture gap exceeding 3cm, previous failed repair, associated perineal fistulas, rectourethral fistulas, periurethral cavities, false passages or an open bladder neck. Destruction or rupture of the posterior urethra is caused mainly by forces that occur during traumatic pelvic fracture. This trauma results in partial or complete rupture of the urethra. A complete rupture often results in destruction of the posterior urethra and may damage the sphincteric structures, while always damaging the neurovascular bundles, which results in impotence and incontinence. Due to prior repeated surgery, patients with complex strictures are often found significant scar tissue formation of the urethra. The problems arise from a lack of the healthy elastic tissue needed to reconstruct the urethra.

2. Assessment

There are a number of different imaging techniques that may be used in imaging the male urethra. The most widespread methods include retrograde urethrography (RUG) and voiding cystourethrography (VCUG). However, other modalities, such as ultrasound, magnetic resonance imaging (MRI), and computed tomography, have been used as adjuncts. Accurate diagnosis of stricture presence, number, location, and length is of paramount importance in planning appropriate treatment. Although RUG and VCUG are often sufficient for this purpose, ultrasound, CT urethrography and MRI can be useful in certain situations, such as the evaluation of spongiofibrosis, rectourethral fistulas and the periurethral tissues.

2.1 Anatomy and symptoms in complex posterior urethral strictures

The posterior urethra consists of a distal membranous segment which, as it traverses the muscular urogenital diaphragm, becomes the narrowest portion of the normal urethra. For a long time, conventional urologic wisdom was that urethral rupture in men occurs at the prostatomembranous junction by a shearing force that avulses the prostatic apex from the urogenital diaphragma. Recent studies suggest that this traditional belief may be a misconception. The urethral sphincter extends from the bladder neck to the perineal membrane (diaphragma urogenitale). The muscular lining and surrounding of the membranous urethra are directly continuous with similar muscle fibers of the prostatic urethra and end abruptly at the perineal membrane. Hence, the weakness may lie in the bulbomembranous junction rather than the prostatomembranous junction at which the posterior urethra is liable to rupture (Fig. 1). More proximally, the prostatic urethra can be seen extending from the bladder neck to the membranous segment. A small longitudinally oriented mound of smooth muscle, the verumontanum, is present along the dorsal aspect of the prostatic urethra and can be seen as a filling defect during fluoroscopic studies. Its distal end marks the proximal aspect of the membranous urethra (3).

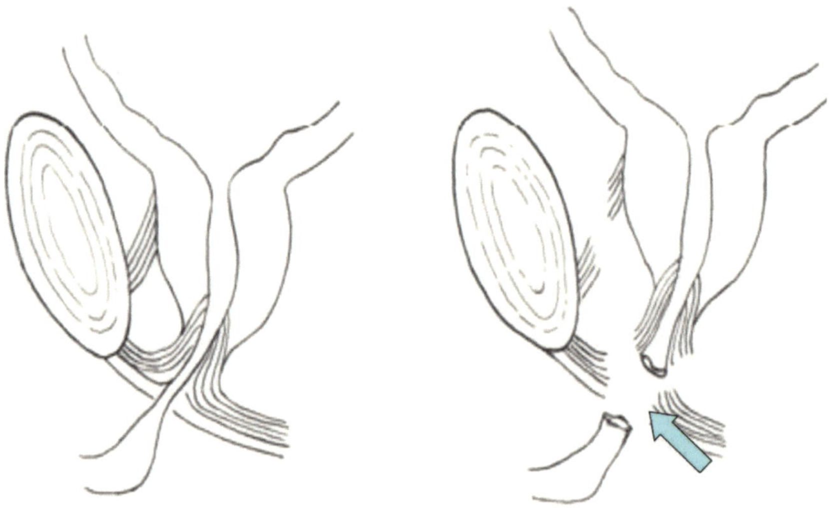

Fig. 1. Bulbomembranous junction (blue arrow), which is the most weakness site in the urethra

Although dysuria is the main symptom in patients with urethral stricture, other special phenomenon can still be noticed in those with complex urethral stricture. In patients with urethrorectal fistula, the most common symptoms are watery stools, urinary incontinence, irritative voiding complaints, and pneumaturia and fecaluria (Fig. 2).

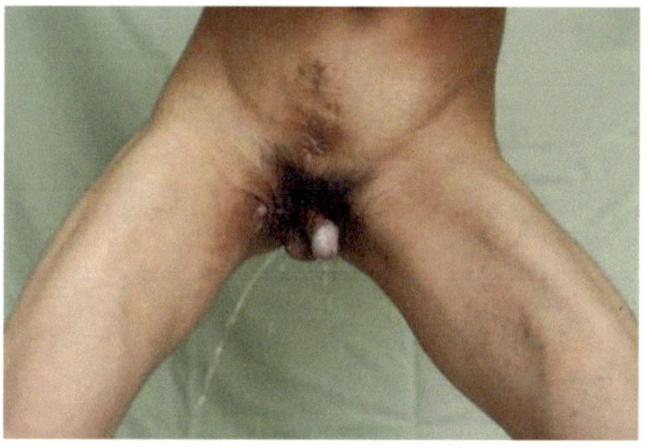

Fig. 2. The main presenting symptom in all cases was urinary leakage through the anus

2.2 Retrograde urethrography and voiding cystourethrography

RUG and VCUG are the most commonly used techniques for male urethral imaging. They are readily available and can be safely and relatively quickly performed. The information they provide is usually sufficient to direct patient care. Serious complications are rare, and the procedure is usually well tolerated by patients.

Useful anatomic landmarks to identify the membranous urethra are the inferior margins of the obturator foramina (Fig. 3). It is particularly important to identify the exact location of the membranous urethra, as this is where the urogenital diaphragm and external sphincter are located. In the trauma setting, injury to the external sphincter may affect urinary continence. Although the posterior urethra is opacified during most examinations, its distention is usually poor after contrast passes through the relatively narrow membranous urethra. To improve visualization of the posterior urethra, the patient can be instructed to void during the examination, distending the posterior segment.

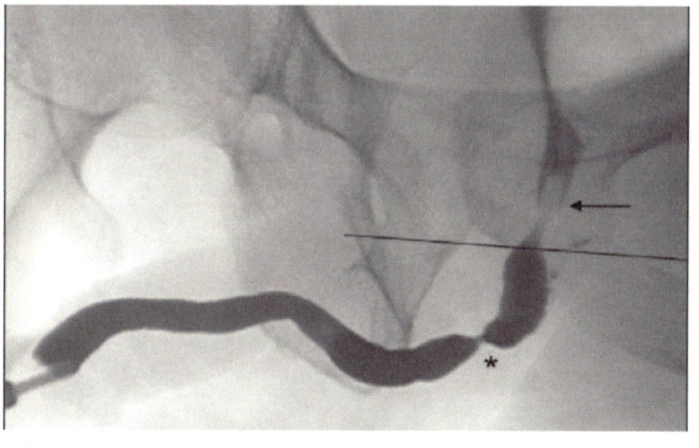

Fig. 3. Bony landmark beneath the inferior margin of the obturator foramina intersects the bulbomembranous junction of the urethra. Arrow head showed a filling defect (verumontanum) in the posterior urethra whose distal end extent to the proximal end of membranous urethra

The VCUG often is performed in conjunction with retrograde urethrography and is especially useful in assessing the posterior urethra. In contrast to the RUG, opening of the bladder neck and distention of the posterior urethra are achieved during VCUG (4).
To perform a VCUG, the bladder is filled with contrast either through the urethra in a retrograde fashion, an indwelling Foley catheter, or a suprapubic catheter. The patient is positioned in much the same way as during a RUG, and instructed to void into a canister. This is more easily accomplished if the fluoroscopy table is tilted upwards so that the patient is in a standing position. Images of the urethra are then obtained during voiding.
It is common to see an apparently long gap between the distal limit of a complete obliteration on ascending (retrograde) urethrogram and the bladder neck on a cystogram (through a suprapubic catheter) (Fig. 4a, b). This doesn't mean that the stricture extends all the way up to the bladder neck, only that the detrusor is unable to contract and open the bladder neck and so allow contrast down to the upper end of the obliteration.
Of course, those technique might be the most common approach for evaluating urethrorectal fistulas (Fig. 5).

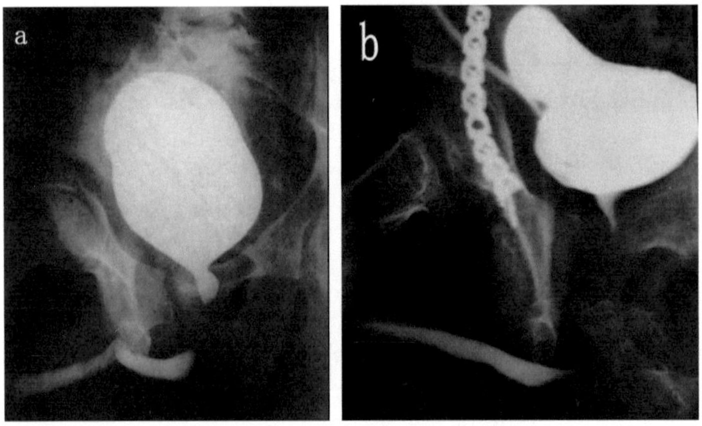

Fig. 4. a,b Combined ascending urethrogram and micturating cystogram helps to define the proximal and distal limits of the stricture

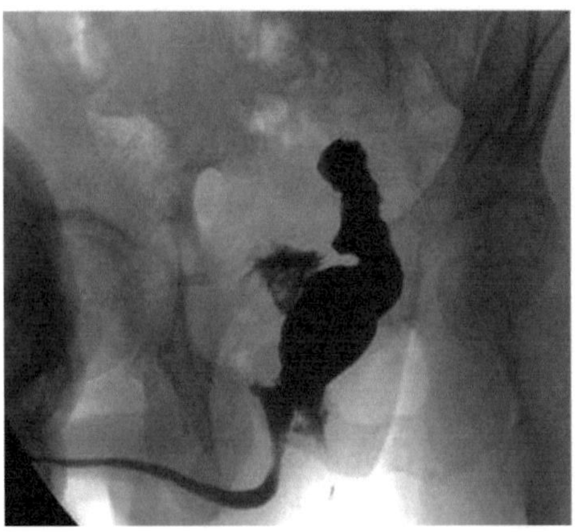

Fig. 5. the preoperative urethrogram showed a connection between urethra and rectum

2.3 Sonourethrography

A less frequently used method of imaging the urethra is sonourethrography, which was introduced in the mid-1980s. It is an accurate tool for the diagnosis and characterization of strictures, particularly of the bulbar urethra. Although less frequently performed, transperineal scans may be obtained to image the posterior urethra (Fig. 6).

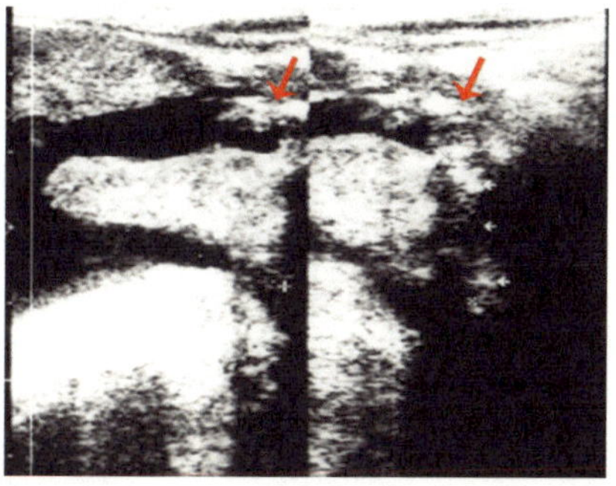

Fig. 6. the site of the posterior urethra stricture from transperineal scans (red arrow)

The advantage of sonourethrography lies in its ability to determine stricture length, especially in the bulbar urethra, with a high degree of accuracy. Because the probe can be oriented along the course of the urethra, there are fewer tendencies to foreshorten the length of a stricture than with RUG. As fibrosis develops, the urethra becomes less distensible compared with the surrounding normal tissues. Areas of periurethral fibrosis appear as hyperechogenicity of the tissues of the spongiosa surrounding the urethra (5). Therefore, sonourethrography may provide information about the soft tissues surrounding the urethra including the degree of spongiofibrosis surrounding the stenotic portions of the lumen (6).

The disadvantages of sonourethrography include its limited availability, cost, limited evaluation of the posterior urethra, and the high level of technical expertise necessary to be able to perform and interpret the exam.

2.4 Magnetic resonance imaging

MRI is infrequently used in the evaluation of the male urethra. In general, the sagittally oriented images are most useful for evaluation the status of urethra. A phased array coil is placed over the perineum, and a small field of view is used. It is not widely available and is an expensive and technically difficult examination to perform. In most cases, little information is gained beyond that provided by other conventional imaging methods. However, MRI can provide useful information in certain clinical situations, particularly in evaluation the situation of posterior urethral trauma and periurethral soft tissues (Fig. 7). The information about the location of the prostate gland and pelvic hematoma may be obtained as well (7,8).

2.5 Voiding CT urethrography

Recently, performing 3-D retrograde CT urethrograms became possible because of the technical developments in multislice CT technology (9). These images allow visualization of the urethra from any angle, without interference caused by the surrounding structures. In urethral stricture disease, the advantage of this technique is becoming more important, especially in documenting the posterior urethra which is located behind bony structures, allowing better visualization of the pathology and better preoperative planning (Fig. 8).

Looking at the 3-D reconstructions of the urethra (or other organs) is almost like performing exploratory.

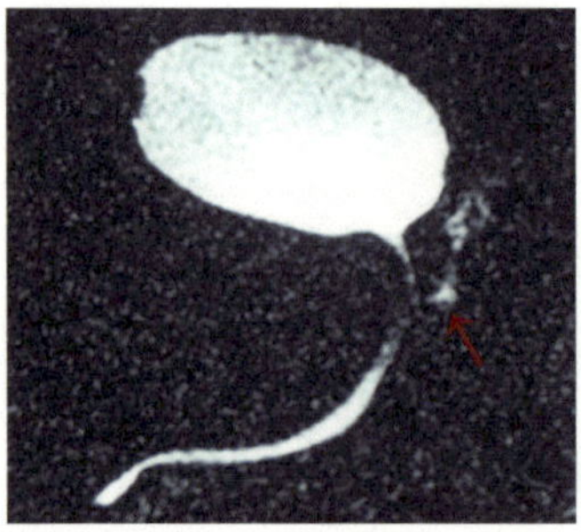

Fig. 7. Sagittal images for evaluation of the posterior urethral stricture and surround tissue

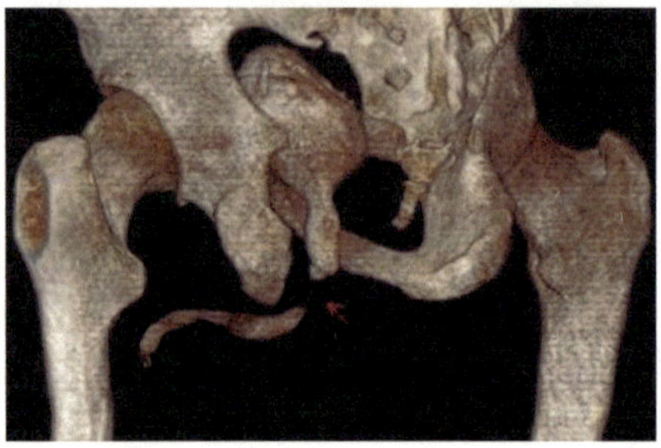

Fig. 8. shows on CTCUG the bladder neck and the proximal part of the prostatic urethra were visualized, the distraction defect (arrow) is about 3cm which was confirmed by the operative finding

CTCUG is also typically fairly sensitive and specific qualitatively for diagnosing a urethrorectal fistula. According to the 3D image obtained from CTCUG, more details about the fistual could be got. It might be the better choice for patients suffered with PFUDDs associated with urethrorectal fistula than other procedures (Fig. 9).

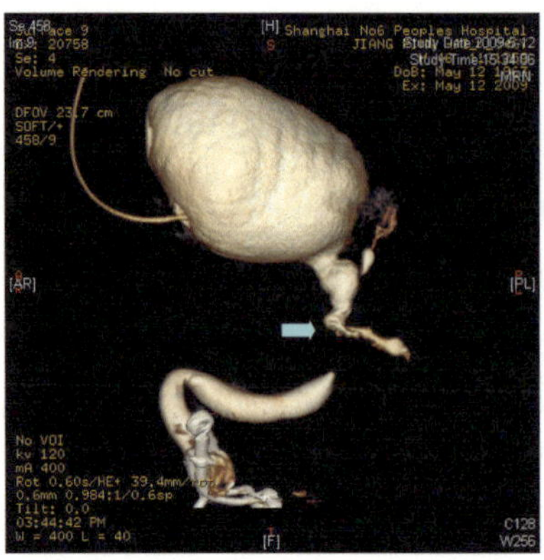

Fig. 9. CTCUG showed a PUDD and urethrorectal fistulas, the defects length is about 4cm, the blue arrow indicate the urethrorectal fistulas

2.6 Urethroscopy

A flexible cystoscopy may be helpful in determining the details of an apparently obstructed or incompetent bladder neck and indeed might be helpful in the overall assessment of the urethra on either side of the obstruction. The 7.5Fr flexible cystoscopy was used to perform urethroscopy under lidocaine jelly 2% intraurethral anesthesia. A flexible cystoscopy is advanced through the urethra until the stricture was encountered (Fig. 10a). Then flexible cystoscopy via a suprapubic cystostomy tract was utilized to locate the proximal segment of a complete traumatic disruption (Fig. 10b). Urethral calculi were identified proximal to the stricture only during urethroscopy (Fig. 10c). The ability to negotiate the stricture visually can provide important information regarding length, density, location in relation to the external sphincter, and any associated pathology before treatment is undertaken. Staging of the stricture adequately in these settings may provide more accurate, and more real-time information than RUG, improving the urologist's ability to select definitive therapy for the patient (10).

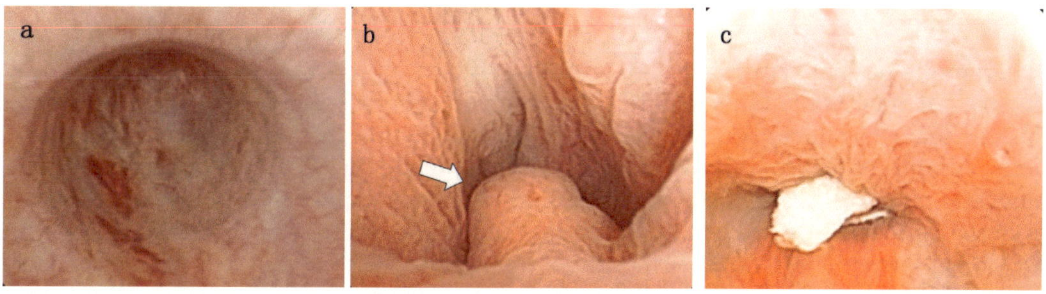

Fig. 10. The image of flexible cystoscopy. a) The obliterative view from the antegrade cystoscopy; b) The obliterative view from the bladder neck, the verumontanum (arrow); c) Calculus can be seen proximal to urethral stricture

Of course, it can be used to determine the degree of damage to the bladder as to capacity and compliance and the location of the fistula in relation to the ureteral orifices and the bladder neck (Fig. 11).

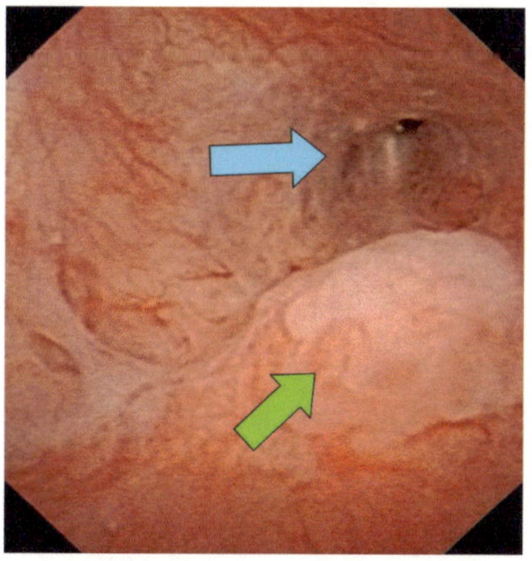

Fig. 11. From the bladder neck, the verumontanum (green arrow) and the urethrorectal fistula (blue arroe) can be seen through a flexible cystoscopy

3. Preparation

The patient is admitted on the day of surgery and requires no special preparation. It is sensible to know the patient's blood group, although blood transfusion is rarely necessary except in complicated cases. It is also sensible to have an up to date urine culture, although prophylactic antibiotics will almost always be given with the pre-medication or with the anesthesia. Since the sound will access to the suprapubic area in order to demonstrate the upper level of the obstruction by palpitation during the course of the procedure, a suprapubic drainage should be performed before surgery.

To patients with urethrorectal fistula, the function of the anal and external urethral sphincters, the presence of a concomitant urethral stricture or bladder neck contracture, the visible and palpable health of the tissue adjacent and near the fistula, and the size and location of the fistula should be determined preoperatively. The fecal and urinary proximal diversion should be performed and the patients nutritionally supplemented.

4. Procedure

4.1 A simple perineal approach

The patient is positioned in standard lithotomy and prepped and draped to give access to the perineum, genitalia, and suprapubic region. A midline perineal skin incision that is bifurcated posteriorly to improve perineal access is made (Fig. 12a). The bulbo-spongiosus muscle is carefully resected to the bulbar urethra and the bulbar urethra is then separated from the perineal body proximally and from the fused corpora cavernosa more distally by division of the raphe that attaches the corpus spongiosum to the fused corpora on its ventral aspect (Fig. 12b). The site of the obliteration of the urethra is easily defined by passing a Foley catheter up the urethra until it can pass and at this site the urethra is transacted (Fig. 13). Scarred tissue and unhealthy urothelium must be dissected off the transected bulbar urethra until the proximal cut end of the bulbar urethra is healthy (11). Occasionally, there is still a lumen through the site of the transection to the healthy posterior urethra above but this is rare. More commonly the posterior urethra above the site of the fibrosis and obliteration is best defined by passing a metal sound through the suprapubic catheter track to help identify the prostatic urethra by palpation through the scar tissue. The verumontanum

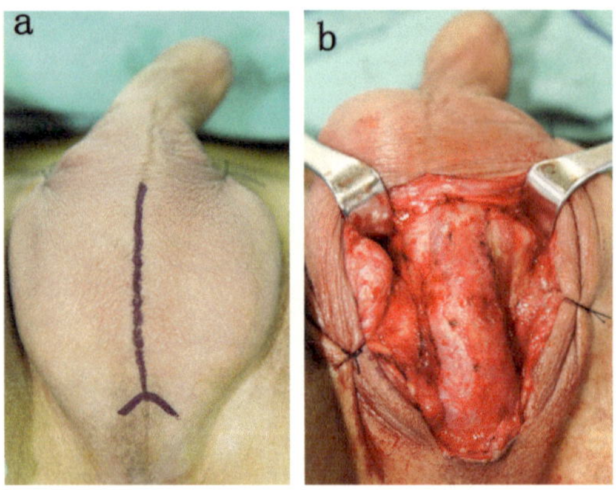

Fig. 12. a) the inverted Y shape incision line in the perineal; b) Exposure and mobilization of the bulbar urethra from within the bulbospongiosus muscle

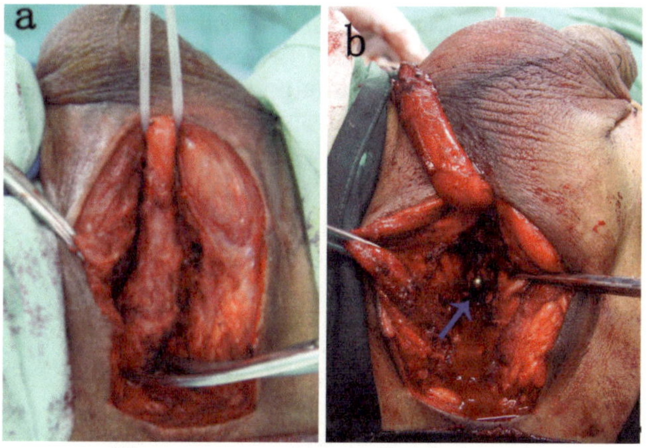

Fig. 13. a) The urethra is then transected through the site of obliteration to free it. b) The sound (blue arrow) indicate the distal end of posterior urethra after transected

is an important landmark for identifying the prostatic urethra and in case of any doubt cystoscopy was performed (12). It is usually then possible to cut through, strictly in the midline, onto the tip of the urethral sound to identify the prostatic urethra and then spatulate it open using six or eight 4/0 Vicryl sutures, which will subsequently be used for the anastomosis. We usually use eight Vicryl sutures at 1:2-, 4:5-, 7: 8-, 10 and 11-o'clock positions. We find that eight sutures is better than six sutures to create a watertight anastomosis. 10 or 12 sutures described by literatures are not suitable for complex posterior urethral cases. It is neither effective nor operational in most cases (Fig. 14).

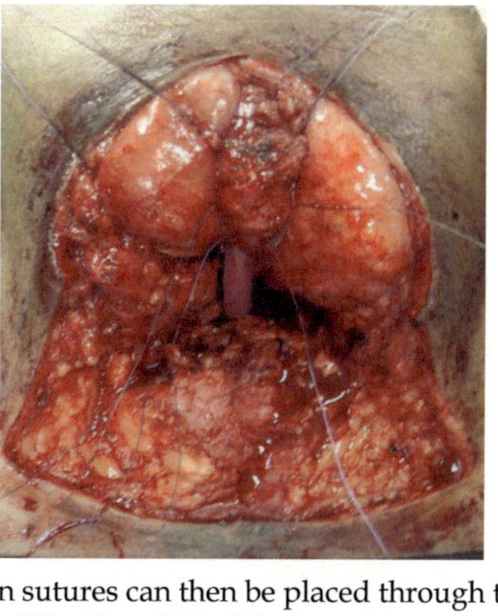

Fig. 14. Eight 4-O polyglactin sutures can then be placed through the full thickness of the proximal urethra at 1:2-, 4:5-, 7:8-, 10 and 11-o'clock positions

The emergency treatment of patients with PFUDD in developing countries is not currently codified and most of these patients have been treated using incorrect procedures that add iatrogenic damage to the trauma. Sometimes careless and repeated urethral dilatation leads to formation of a urethral false passage(s), resulting in infection and incontinence (Fig. 15).

For those patients with post-traumatic posterior urethral strictures compliance with urethral false passage, it also can be effectively treated by trans-perineal approach. It is important that the urethral false passage and the real urethra should be distinguished during surgery (13). When the catheterization procedure is carried out crudely, urethral false passage is likely to form and can be subsequently mistaken for the real urethra. In our country, emergency treatment was carried out at the local primary hospital and included catheterization. Most of patients were treated for urethral realignment and the posterior urethral scar tissue electrovaporization and electroresection procedure were performed. We discovered a lot of urethral false passage formation from bladder to urinary meatus (Fig. 16).

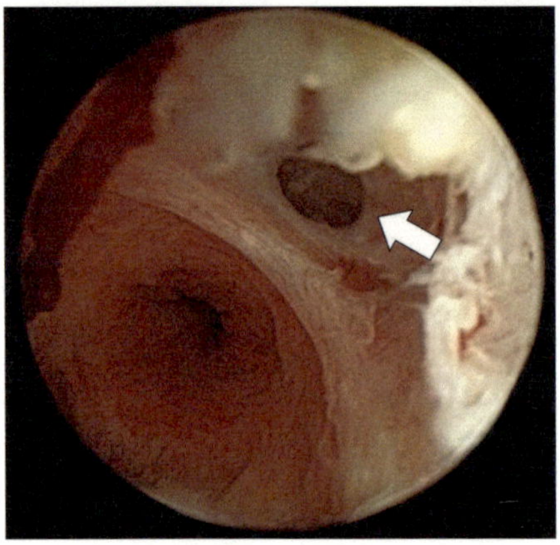

Fig. 15. Careless and repeated urethral dilatation leads to formation of a urethral false passage (arrow), a strictured area with a fibrous-appearing band

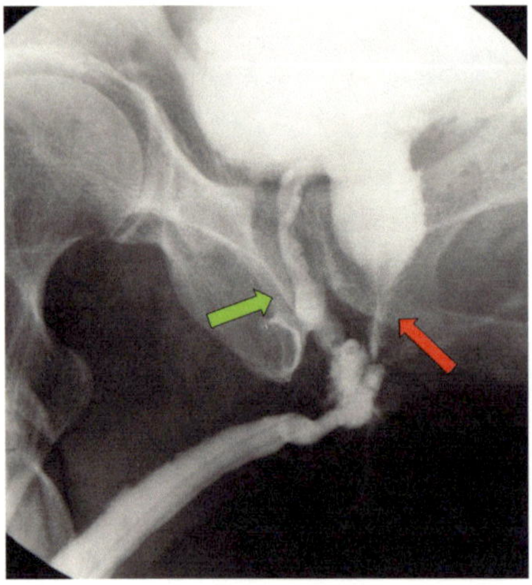

Fig. 16. Pre-operative urography for the patient. The passage marked with a green arrow is the false passage from bladder to urinary meatus. The passage marked with a red arrow is the real urethra

In the circumstances of suspectful a false passage, we usually open the bladder and then put the finger in to the bladder neck for identifying the right path or a flexible cystoscopy was used to obverse the verumontanum. At this point the verumontanum should be clearly visible within the posterior urethra, which is a useful point for distinguishing the urethra proper from a false passage. The false passage was resected and the stub was ligated. Meanwhile, we resected the scar tissue of the real urethra and undertook end-to-end anastomosis.

4.2 A transperineal inferior pubectomy approach

More usually there is a longer defect and, therefore, some tension between the two ends when they are drawn together for anastomosis in this way. If this is the case, then a transperineal inferior pubectomy will be necessary to reduce the length of the defect and produce a tension-free anastomosis (14-16). This manoeuvre is mainly designed to reduce the natural curve of the bulbar urethra in order to achieve a tension-free anastomosis.

The first step is separation of the fused corpora cavernosa as they lie over the pubic symphysis such that the bulbar urethra comes to lie between them (Fig. 17). The corporal bodies are separated, beginning at the level of the crus and progressing distally along a relatively avascular midline plane for approximately 4 to 5 cm. Further distal separation is usually not possible due to the more intimate connection between the corporal bodies. This separation allows the urethra to lie between the separated corporal bodies, thereby shortening the distance to the anastomosis (17).

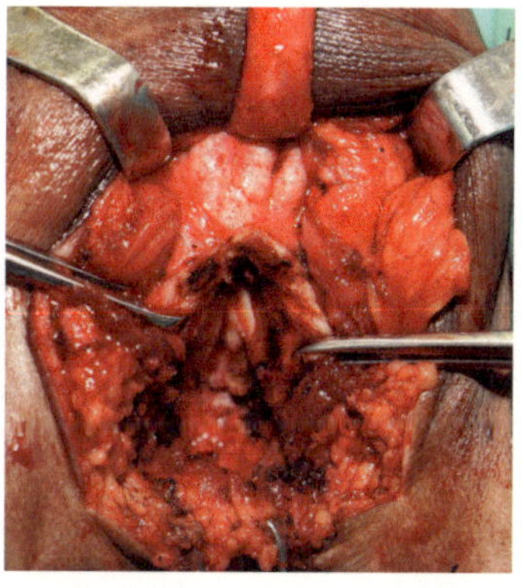

Fig. 17. Separation of the fused corpora cavernosa as they lie over the pubic symphysis

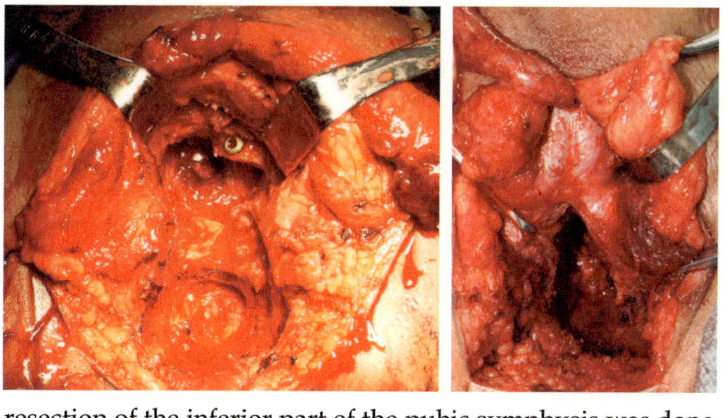

Fig. 18. Wedge resection of the inferior part of the pubic symphysis was done

The next step is removal of the inferior margin of the pubic symphysis (Fig. 18). If tension still exists, the dorsal penile vessels are displaced laterally or ligated and a wedge of bone is excised from the inferior aspect of the pubis using an osteotome and bone rongeurs, the wedge being large enough to allow the urethra be redirected cephalad to lie within the groove, resulting in an additional 1 to 2 cm of apparent urethral length. This maneuver also exposes the anteriorly displaced prostate, thereby facilitating the anastomosis.

The final maneuver is rerouting the urethra around the corporal body through a bony defect created by further pubectomy, shortening the distance to anastomosis by up to an additional 2 cm. For this maneuver one corporal body is circumferentially mobilized at or just proximal to the suspensory ligament. The dissection is carried out away from the surface of the corporal body to avoid injury to neurovascular structures (Fig. 19a). Care must be taken during opening of the dorsal aspect to avoid damage to the deep dorsal vein of the penis in the midline and, particularly, to the dorsal artery and nerve of the penis on either side. This maneuver does not cause significant penile torsion or chordee (Fig. 19b).

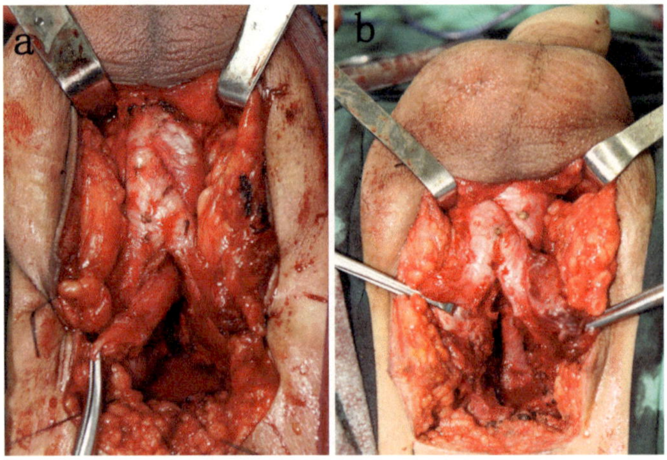

Fig. 19. a) reroute the distal end of urethra. b) the anastomosed urethra after reroute

By combining the two techniques, sectioning the cavernosa septum and chiseling off the lower margin of the pubis, the operative field could be clearly exposed and the path of the anastomotic urethra could be shortened. Then, the penile urethra can hide in the gap, which shortens the distance between the anterior and posterior urethra by about 2-3 cm. Therefore, tension-free anastomosis can be achieved, and postoperative penile shortening caused by excessive dissociation of the distal urethra can be prevented.

From 1990 to 2010, we have used this technique to treat nearly 2200 patients with complex posterior urethral strictures, ranging from 3.5 to 5.0 cm in length. Based on our experience, in cases of a high-lying prostate, the anastomosis may remain under tension. To address this, the proximal corporeal bodies can be separated at the level of the crus and dissected along the relatively avascular midline plane for about 4 to 5 cm. This technique can achieve about 1 to 2 cm of apparent urethral lengthening. We found it was not necessary to re-route the urethra around the corporeal body to provide additional length in those patients.

Having completed the anastomosis, a 16Fr or 18Fr silicone Foley urethral catheter is passed up into the bladder, and suprapubic catheter should be replaced as well. The wound is then closed in layers taking care to obliterate all the dead space as far as possible to reduce the risk of hematoma formation. A wound drain should be left in place for 2 or 3days to prevent the accumulation of any hematoma.

For treating the posterior urethral stricture asssociated with rectourethral fistulas, inferior pubectomy approach can be selected based on the complexity and etiology of the lesion (18,19). Young and Stone in 1917 first used a perineal exposure with a wide dissection, separating the rectum from the urethra and prostate, dividing the fistula after extensive rectal mobilization and performing rectal excision followed by a colocutaneous anastomosis. Goodwin et al modified this procedure in 1958 by using an anterior perineal space dissection, closing the defects and interposing a levator ani muscle successfully in patients with acquired rectourethral fistulas. Subsequent interest in the use of the interposition flaps has further enhanced the successful outcome of patients managed by the perineal approach and should be routinely employed in the complex cases where a wide separation is required and sufficiently large muscle flaps are interposed (20-22). The combined abdomino-perineal approach provides good exposure and was most suitable for refractory, complex, posterior, long-segment urethral strictures and large rectourethral fistulas located far from the anus. This technique may work well in cases where there is excessive perineal scar tissue or for patients for whom a prior perineal procedure was unsuccessful. However, we do not recommend this technique as the first-line approach in these patients, especially in pediatric cases. The transperineal–inferior pubic approach, which fully exposes the space behind the pubis and does not lead to pelvic instability, has a lower incidence of postoperative complications. Therefore, it may be appropriate as a first-line procedure in those patients (23).

The procedure is performed with the patient in a moderately dorsal lithotomy position utilizing an inverted 'U'shaped incision from mid-perineum to ischial tuberosities. A midline dissection above the external sphincter is maintained without a lateral or posterior extension separating the rectum, prostate, and subvesical surface up to the peritoneum. The dissection was done at the recto-urethral septum up to a level at least 3 cm above the fistula (Fig. 20). This type of dissection will prevent injury to the innervation of the rectum, anal sphincter, and penile corpora, thereby preserving potency and urinary continence, and should also be used in the smaller fistulas of surgical or traumatic origin. The fistula core was dissected to the rectum and excised (Fig. 21). These defects can be repaired by primary closure with direct approximation of the urethral side with one layer of interrupted 4-0 Monocryl (Fig. 22).

The key to success in this repair is interposition of a viable tissue flap between rectum and urethra. Here, we suggested using gracilis flap in this kind of operation. It has been widely used for the reconstruction of vaginal, vulvoperineal or inguinal defects to fill perineal skin defects created by a variety of surgical procedures, such as in the treatment of Paget's disease and penile and urethral cancer (24,25). The advantage of gracilis muscle is that the flap is close to the defect and good blood supply from the branches of the profunda femoralis artery. The complication rate after the muscle transposition is generally minimal.

The gracilis muscle was mobilized and released from its insertions (Fig. 23). The flap was rotated and the distal end was brought to the perineal area through a subcutaneous tunnel (Fig. 24). The muscle was laid between the rectum and the urethra and was fixed at least 3 cm above the fistula site (Fig. 25). All patients underwent fecal diversion, ileostomy or colostomy. Stomal closure was performed after voiding cystourethrography or evaluation under anesthesia and endoscopic demonstration of a healed fistula. Patient outcomes were assessed after surgical repair.

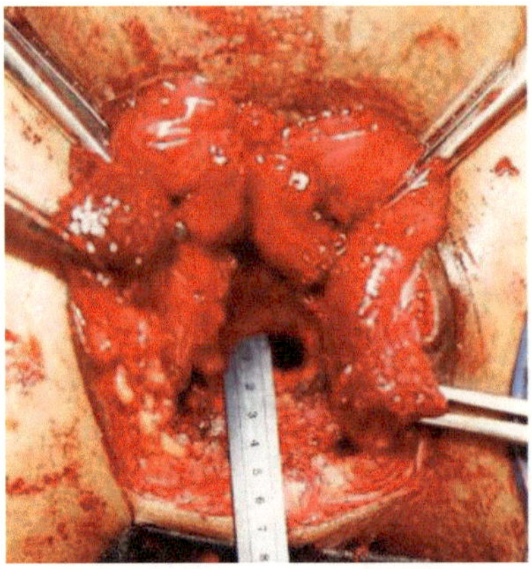

Fig. 20. The dissection is undertaken to divide the fistula tract and reach cephalad to noninflamed tissue

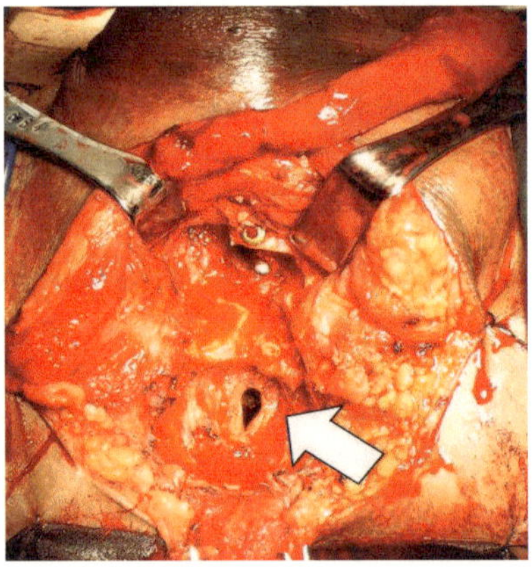

Fig. 21. Intra-operative view after perineal incision and dissection at the recto-urethral septum with a rectourethral fistula (arrow)

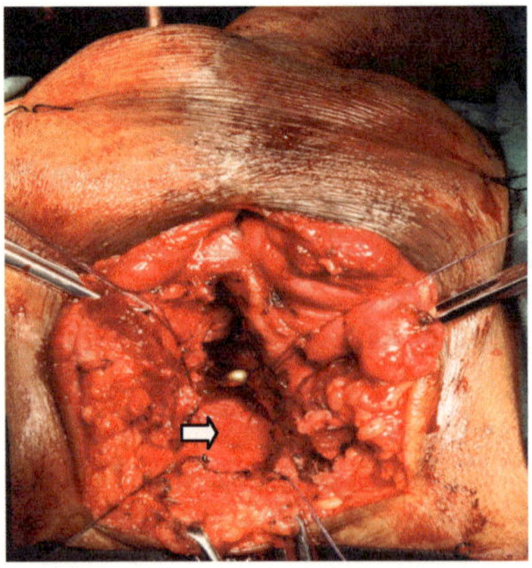

Fig. 22. Closure of the rectal portion of the fistula was performed (arrow)

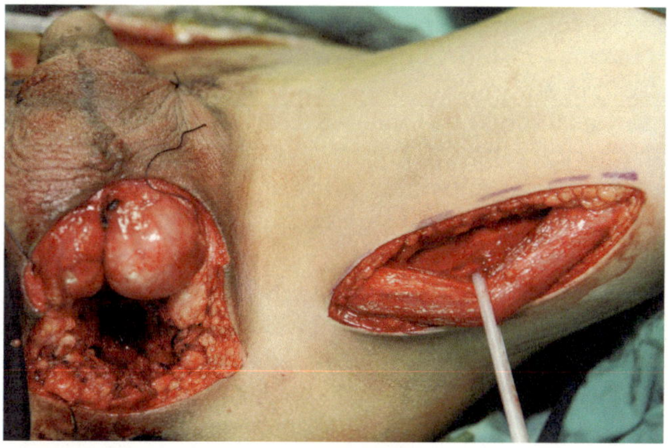

Fig. 23. Release and mobilisation of the gracilis muscle

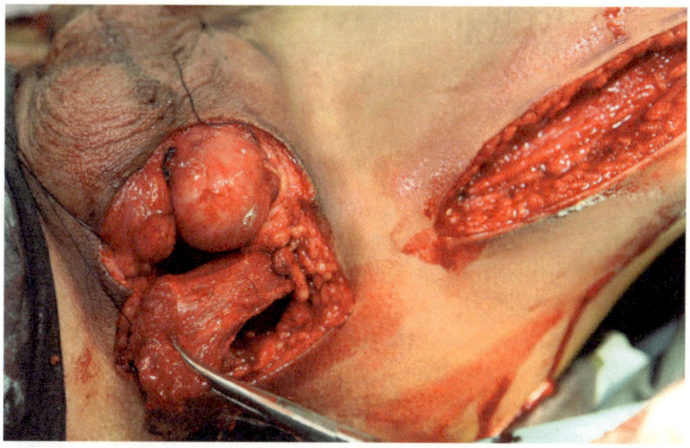

Fig. 24. The flap was rotated and the distal end was brought to the perineal area through a subcutaneous tunnel

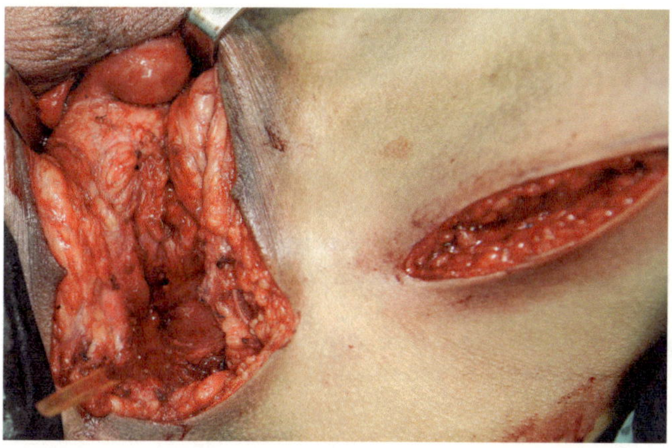

Fig. 25. Inset of the rotated flap between the rectum and the urethra

We emphasize the need for bowel diversion before attempting reconstruction. Moreover, important technical features include meticulous hemostasis, tension-free primary repair of the rectum after dissection and mobilization to a level of at least 3 cm above the fistula site and a tension-free transposition of the well-vascularized gracilis muscle. The results of our study have shown that recto-urethral fistula closure using the perineal approach with pedicle gracilis muscle interposition has a low morbidity and a high success rate. Nevertheless, the gracilis muscle interposition is an option for treatment of these complex fistulas (26).

4.3 The combined transpubic- perineal approach

The overwhelming majority of PFUDDs can be repaired successfully through the trans-perineal or inferior pubectomy approach as noted above, as defects as long as 10cm are amenable to repair. Only occasionally is it necessary to use an combined transpubic with perineal approach when there is a chronic periurethral cavity, bladder-neck injury, or some other coincidental problem which requires that approach or otherwise when the prostatic urethra is inaccessible from below, or in a severe bulbar crush injury leaving only the distal bulbar urethra intact or those patients who have failed a prior repair (16).

The combined transpubic- perineal approach involves both perineal and retropubic exposure of the urethra and prostate with removal of a segment of pubic bone to facilitate exposure. It was usually suggested in pediatric patients due to their narrow and deep pelvic outlet along with the abdominal location of bladder, which often makes a perineal approach suboptimal for adequate expouse (27,28). In some cases, their bladder neck might be non-functional either as a result of unrecognized or unrepaired injury at the time of pelvic fracture, prior resection or prostatectomy, or simply because of fixation in the periprostatic retropubic scar. In such cases, a transpubic- perineal approach has been suggested (17,29). Furthermore, the periurethral cavity formed from a liquefied pelvic hematoma can also be treated thorough this approach (30).

This approach was first performed by Pierce in 1962 and his approach allowed excellent visualization of the vesical neck, entire posterior urethra and the urogenital diaphragm. Waterhouse et al utilized this approach with a few modifications. He described excising an entire anterior wedge of pubis using a Gigli saw (31,32). Inferior wedge pubectomy will have been completed perineally, and this—combined with retropubic bone removal—will provide wide anterior access, which facilitates anastomosis and access to the pelvic floor to manage the complicating features that were the indication for this approach (33). We think that entire wedge pubectomy or inferior wedge pubectomy should be selected based on the complexity of local condition, such as surrounding scar tissue, the degree of exposure. Their technique combined exposing the periprostatic space by pubectomy followed by anterior urethral mobilization by a perineal approach (34,35).

In details, the patient was placed in standard lithotomy position. The thighs were abducted and the knees flexed providing access to the perineum. A midline subumbilical abdominal incision was made and carried well down to the root of the penis (Fig. 26a). The retropubic space and a plane must be developed between the sumphysis and the underlying prostate and bladder. A Gigli saw is then passed on a right angle clamp from the retropubic space below the lower border of the pubic. The Gigli saw was pulled well laterally and the pubic was sawed through. A similar procedure was then performed on the other side and the wedge of the bone was removed approximately 2 cm on each side of the symphsis pubic (Fig. 26b,c). Identification of the proximal urethra beneath the fibrous tissue was done using a boogie passed through the bladder neck under direct vision or a finger can be used to help direct the retropubic dissection and avoid damage the bladder neck (36).

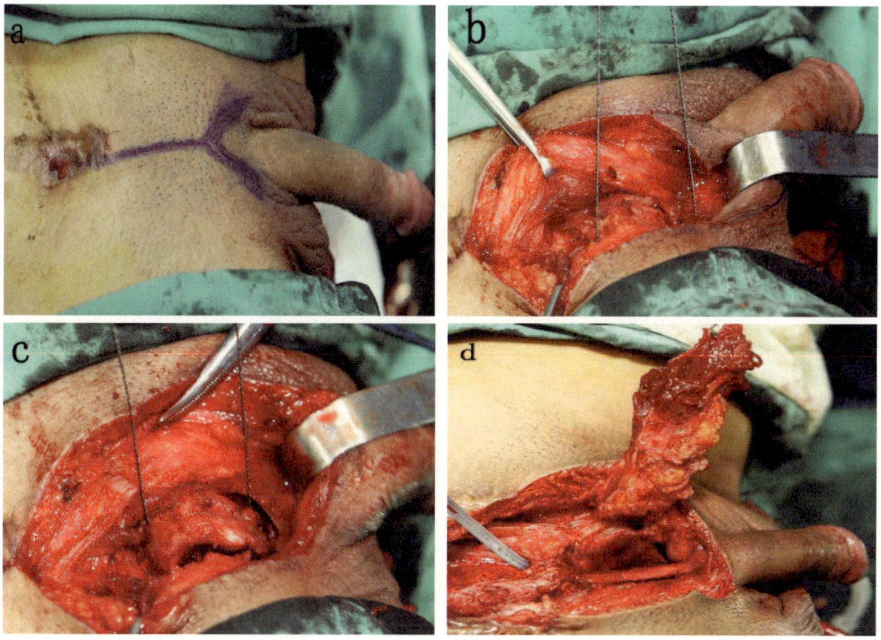

Fig. 26. Process of combined abdominal-perineal approach for urethroplasty was showed. a) a vertical midline incision was made and carried well down to the root of the penis b) a Gigli saw is then passed on a right angle clamp from the retropubic space c) a Gigli saw is then passed on a left angle clamp from the retropubic space. d) removal of a wedge of pubic bone and allowed a simultaneous perineal approach for distal urethral mobilization end-to-end urethroplasty was performed

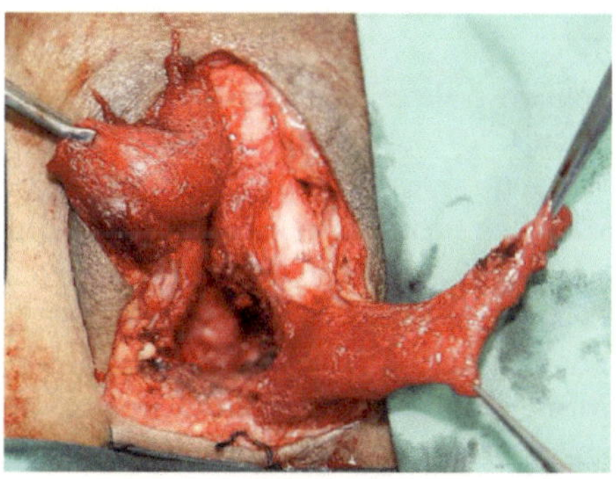

Fig. 27. The dartos muscle from the scrotum was used to supports urethral anastomosis

A midline perineal incision was also made to expose the anterior urethra. The distal urethra was mobilized distally up to glans and proximally up to triangular ligament and was transected at this level. The mobilized urethra was passed through an incision made in intercrural septum. End-to-end urethroplasty was performed over a 16Fr silicon catheter using six or eight interrupted 4-0 absorbable sutures (Fig. 26d). The dead space around the anastomosis needs to be obliterated by various methods including: mobilization of the cremester fascia or dartos muscle from the scrotum; pedicled omentum; sliding a pedicled gracilis muscle belly from the medial aspect of the thigh, or by vertical rectus abdominis muscle flap (Fig. 27). A surprapubic catheter was inserted through the bladder dome. Retropubic space suction drain was then placed.

5. Postoperative follow-up

A urethrogram with catheter should be arranged in each patients 2 weeks after operation. All patients should be followed up for 6 months or so later. And urinary flowmetry ,the ascending urethrogram, micturating cystogram will be repeated during the follow-up .

6. Complications

6.1 Failure of repair

The most common presentation of a recurrent stricture is that the patient runs into trouble within hours or days of having their postoperative catheter removed. This is because such problems are as a result of ischemia of the anastomosis because the blood supply is insufficient to sustain adequate vascularity of the anastomosis, fibrotic tissue was left behind. More commonly, tension anastomosis during operation may lead to the recurrence. If the procedure was performed technically competently then almost always the patients who show this early failure also have complete erectile dysfunction supporting the concept that this recurrent stricture is vasculogenic and ischaemic in origin. In such cases, the suprapubic catheter must be replaced and the patient must wait another three months and the procedure is repeated.

6.2 Erectile dysfunction and incontinence

In many patients with complex posterior strictures, stricture resection and bulboprostatic anastomosis yielded good results of operation. Since those strictures are usually the result of severe pelvic trauma in which the urethra is disrupted from the pelvic floor, and during which neurovascular bundles are torn, 30%–50% of the patients already have erectile dysfunction prior to the bulboprostatic anastomosis. Complication of erectile dysfunction is generally related to the original injury rather than the procedure itself. Our previous study showed that the neurogenic factors may be the principal etiology of organic impotence associated with urethral injury. The type of pelvic fracture, in particular fractures associated with the pubic diastasis, is particularly important. The location of stricture is also a risk factor for loss of potency (37,38). On the other hand, the erectile function will recovery in some patients within 6 months postoperatively, which is due to the decompression of erectile nerve bundles. Therefore, intimate following up after operation is absolutely necessary in those patient. Further treatment of impotence is only considered in those patients suffered with erectile dysfunction for a long period of time after the urethroplasty. There may also be postoperative incontinence due to surgery-related damage to the intrinsic sphincter organ when the bladder neck is incompetent, when the bladder neck is involved in the primary trauma. This complication can be avoided by a carefully assessment before surgery.

7. References

[1] Barbagli G. History and evolution of transpubic urethroplasty: a lesson for young urologists in training. *Eur Urol* 2007; 52: 1290–1292

[2] Kulkarni SB, Barbagli G, Kulkarni JS, Romano G, Lazzeri M. Posterior urethral stricture after pelvic fracture urethral distraction defects in developing and developed countries, and choice of surgical technique. J Urol. 2010; 183:1049-1054.
[3] Pavlica P, Barozzi L, Menchi I. Imaging of male urethra. Eur Radiol 2003; 13:1583-1596.
[4] Kawashima A, Sandler CM, Wasserman NF, LeRoy AJ, King BF Jr, Goldman SM. Imaging of urethral disease: a pictorial review. Radiographics 2004; 24 Suppl 1:S195-216.
[5] Choudhary S, Singh P, Sundar E, Kumar S, Sahai A. A comparison of sonourethrography and retrograde urethrography in evaluation of anterior urethral strictures. Clin Radiol 2004; 59:736-742.
[6] Mitterberger M, Christian G, Pinggera GM, Bartsch G, Strasser H, Pallwein L, et al. Gray scale and color Doppler sonography with extended field of view technique for the diagnostic evaluation of anterior urethral strictures. J Urol 2007; 177:992-996; discussion 997.
[7] Gallentine ML, Morey AF. Imaging of the male urethra for stricture disease. Urol Clin North Am 2002; 29:361-372.
[8] Ryu J, Kim B. MR imaging of the male and female urethra. Radiographics 2001; 21:1169-1185.
[9] El-Kassaby AW, Osman T, Abdel-Aal A, Sadek M, Nayef N.Dynamic three-dimensional spiral computed tomographic cysto-urethrography: a novel technique for evaluating post-traumatic posterior urethral defects. BJU Int. 2003; 92:993-996
[10] Figueroa JC, Hoenig DM. Use of 7.5F flexible pediatric cystoscope in the staging and management of urethral stricture disease. Joul Endourology. 2004; 18:119-121.
[11] Mundy AR. Anastomotic urethroplasty. BJU Int 2005; 96:921-944.
[12] Mundy AR. Transperineal bulbo-prostatic anastomotic urethroplasty. World J Urol 1998; 16: 164-170.
[13] Singla M, Jha MS, Muruganandam K, Srivastava A, Ansari MS, Mandhani A, et al. Posttraumatic posterior urethral strictures in children--management and intermediate-term follow-up in tertiary care center. Urology 2008, 72:540-543; discussion 543-544
[14] Fu Q, Zhang J, Sa YL, Jin SB, Xu YM. Transperineal bulboprostatic anastomosis in patients with simple traumatic posterior urethral strictures: A retrospective study from a referral urethral center. Urology, 2009; 74(5):1132-6.
[15] Fu Q, Xu YM, Zhang J, Jin SB, Sa YL. Use of anastomotic urethroplasty with partial pubectomy for posterior urethral obliteration injuries: 10 years experience. World J Urol 2009; 27:695-699.
[16] Andrich, DE, Mundy AR. What is the Best Technique for Urethroplasty? Eur Urol 2008; 54:1031-1041
[17] Webster GD, Guralnick ML. Reconstruction of posterior urethral disruption. Urol Clin North Am 2002; 29:429-441.
[18] Zmora O, Potenti FM, Wexner SD, Pikarsky AJ, Efron JE, Nogueras JJ,et al. Gracilis muscle transposition for iatrogenic rectourethral fistula. Ann Surg 2003; 237:483-487.
[19] Lane BR, Stein DE, Remzi FH, Strong SA, Fazio VW, Angermeier KW. Management of radiotherapy induced rectourethral fistula. J Urol 2006; 175:1382-1387; discussion 1387-1388.
[20] Ulrich D, Roos J, Jakse G, Pallua N. Gracilis muscle interposition for the treatment of recto-urethral and rectovaginal fistulas: a retrospective analysis of 35 cases. Journal of Plastic, Reconstructive & Aesthetic Surgery 2009:62, 352-356.

[21] Gupta G, Kumar S, Kekre NS, Gopalakrishnan G. Surgical management of rectourethral fistula. Urology 2008; 71:267-271.
[22] Joshi HM, Vimalachandran D, Heath RM, Rooney PS. Management of iatrogenic recto-urethral fistula by transanal rectal flap advancement. Colorectal Dis 2010.
[23] Xu YM, Sa YL, Fu Q, Zhang J, Jin SB. Surgical Treatment of 31 Complex Traumatic Posterior Urethral Strictures Associated with Urethrorectal Fistulas. Eur Urol 2010; 57:514-520.
[24] Rabau M, Zmora O, Tulchinsky H, Gur E, Goldman G. Recto-vaginal/urethral fistula: repair with gracilis muscle transposition. Acta Chir Iugosl 2006; 53:81-84.
[25] Osawa S, Nishimura T, Akimoto M, Abe H, Hamasaki T, Kuroda S. Repair of a fistula between the bladder and the perineal skin by femoral gracilis flap interposition. Int J Urol 2001; 8:80-82.
[26] Ulrich D, Roos J, Jakse G, Pallua N. Gracilis muscle interposition for the treatment of recto-urethral and rectovaginal fistulas: a retrospective analysis of 35 cases. J Plast Reconstr Aesthet Surg 2009; 62:352-356.
[27] Kizer WS, Armenakas NA, Brandes SB, Cavalcanti AG, Santucci RA, Morey AF. Simplified reconstruction of posterior urethral disruption defects: limited role of supracrural rerouting. J Urol 2007; 177:1378-1381; discussion 1381-1382.
[28] Zhang J, Xu YM, Qiao Y, Jin SB, Wu DL, Gu BJ. An evaluation of surgical approaches for posterior urethral distraction defects in boys. J Urol 2006; 176:292-295; discussion 295.
[29] Iselin CE, Webster GD. The significance of the open bladder neck associated with pelvic fracture urethral distraction defects. J Urol 1999; 162:347-351.
[30] Al-Rifaei MA, Zaghloul S, Al-Rifaei AM. Bulboprostatic anastomotic urethroplasty with preservation of potency: anatomical study, operative approach and clinical results. Scand J Urol Nephrol 2005; 39:163-168.
[31] Waterhouse K, Abrahams JI, Gruber H , Hackett RE, Patil UB, Peng BK. The transpubic approach to the lower urinary tract. J Urol 1973; 109: 486–490.
[32] Turner-Warwick R. Complex traumatic posterior urethral strictures. J Urol 1977; 118: 564–574.
[33] Pratap A, Agrawal CS, Tiwari A, Bhattarai BK, Pandit RK, Anchal N. Complex posterior urethral disruptions: management by combined abdominal transpubic perineal urethroplasty. J Urol 2006; 175: 1751–1754, discussion 1754.
[34] Gupta NP, Mishra S, Dogra, PN, Yadav R, Seth A, Kumar R.Transpubic urethroplasty for complex posterior urethral strictures: A single center experience. Urol Int 2009; 83:22–26.
[35] Koraitim MM. Transpubic urethroplasty revisited: total, superior, or inferior pubectomy? Urology 2010; 75:691-694.
[36] Webster GD, MacDiarmid SA. Posterior urethral reconstruction. In: Webster GD, Kirby R, King L, Goldwasser B, editors. Reconstructive urology. Boston: Blackwell Scientific; 1993. Chapter 49.
[37] Feng C, Xu YM, Yu JJ, Fei XF, Chen L. Risk factors for erectile dysfunction in patients with urethral strictures secondary to blunt trauma. J Sex Med 2008; 5:2656-2661.
[38] Morey AF, McAninch JW. Reconstruction of posterior urethral disruption injuries: outcome analysis in 82 patients. J Urol 1997; 157:506-510.

8

Oral Mucosa Graft: An Ideal Substitute for Urethroplasty

Maged Ragab and Hossam Haroun
Tanta University, Tanta
EGYPT

1. Introduction

Urethroplasty is both an art and science. The fact that over 200 different types of repair have been reported in the literatures confirms that it is a difficult surgery with many complications and frequently inadequate cosmetic and functional results. (1)
There are two main principles of urethroplasty:

- Anastomotic technique.
- Tissue transfer.

The use of vascularized local penile or preputial skin has been the mainstay of urethral reconstruction for a long time. Lacking of penile and preputial skin necessitated the search for new sources for tissue transfer. Resurgence of the use of free grafts for anterior urethral stricture reconstruction has renewed the search for the ideal urethral substitute. (1)
Since 1909, a large variety of free extra genital graft tissues had been described in the literature for substitution urethroplasty e.g. ureter (2), tunica vaginalis (3), full thickness extragenital skin (4), and bladder mucosa. (5)
For 100 years, oral mucosa had variously been utilized as a free graft in reconstructive plastic surgery. (6) The first report on the application of oral mucosa as a substitute for conjunctiva dated back to 1873 when Stellwag Von Carion used the lip mucosa to treat conjunctival defects. (6)
It is generally accepted that Humby, a plastic surgeon, first proposed and reported the use of buccal mucosa in urethral surgery for hypospadias repair in 1941. (7) Whether owing to lack of suitable antibiotic prophylaxis or technical factors, the technique did not gain acceptance or widespread use at that time until almost 50 years later. Current enthusiasm for the technique was promoted by Duckett 1986, (8) Burger and associates 1992 (9), Dessanti and colleagues 1992 (10) and Elkasaby et al. (11)
In the following years, numerous reports had described successful use of buccal mucosal graft in the repair of urethral defects associated with previously failed hypospadias surgery and those associated with urethral stricture. (12-19) Nowadays, buccal mucosa has become the mainstay of these tissue transfer techniques. (13)
In February 2006, Simonato et al. (20) described the results of the first pilot study on the use of the tongue as an alternative donor site for graft urethroplasty with good functional and aesthetic results. (20) One year later in a dog model, Song et al (21) investigated the feasibility of the LMG urethroplasty. Macroscopic examination of the graft showed no ulceration, calcification, strictures, diverticulae or fistula formation. The junction between

the graft and the normal urethra was discernible by its gross appearance, and the LMGs were tightly incorporated into the urethral walls. (21)
Since then, numerous reports for the use of the lingual mucosa for urethroplasty were published in the last 5 years (16, 21-30) emphasizing Simonato's conclusion that the mucosa of the tongue is a safe and effective graft material in the armamentarium for urethral reconstruction with potential minor risks of donor site complications. (27)

2. Histology of the Oral mucosa

The unique structure of the oral mucosa allows it to be an excellent graft material. (31) The location of the buccal mucosa is limited to the outer vestibule of the oral cavity, which is the space and structure from the teeth to the cheek inside the mouth. Buccal mucosa is freely mobile, loose and compliant. It is 500um thick and a nonkeratinized stratified squameous epithelium consisting of four layers; the stratum basale, stratum spinosum, stratum intermedium and stratum superficiale. (31)
The stratum basale or germinative layer is the basal layer of the epithelium that rests against the basement membrane and provides the progenitor cells for cellular division. It is two to three cells thick and includes melanocytes, antigen-presenting langerhans cells, sensory Merkel cells and lymphocytes. Its rapid mitotic division provides a fast turnover rate, with only 25 days required for all layers of the buccal mucosa to be replaced. (32)
The stratum spinosum is the next layer, which provides the intercellular bridges that give the buccal mucosa the prickle look under light microscopy. The outer two layers stratum intermedium and stratum superficiale are difficult to delineate from each other. These two layers, however, are unique in that they are more firmly attached to each other, providing excellent barrier protection. (32)
The lamina propria of the buccal mucosa is rich in collagen and elastin. Elastin fibers are more numerous in the buccal mucosa than in other tissues, allowing the buccal mucosa to recoil after stretching. The lamina propria further provides long, slender papillary invaginations into the epithelium and loose collagen fibers and loops of capillaries from which the epithelium gets its blood supply. The web like reticular layer of the lamina propria holds the vasculature and nerves of the buccal mucosa. The lamina propria is thin compared with bladder mucosa and skin, which facilitates inosculation and neovascularization. The line between the submucosa and the lamina propria is difficult to delineate. The submucosa, which is firmly attached to the underlying buccinator muscle, is also rich in collagen and elastin, which makes the tissue easy to handle and durable. There are also minor salivary and sebaceous glands. A major salivary gland duct (Stensen's duct) from the parotid gland pierces the buccinators muscle opposite the maxillary second molar bilaterally. (31)
The arterial blood supply to the buccal mucosa originates from the facial artery, the buccal artery, the posterior superior alveolar artery, and the anterior superior alveolar artery. These perforate the buccinator muscle to supply the buccal mucosa. Sensory input for the buccal mucosa is carried through the trigeminal nerve, and buccinators motor function is supplied by cranial nerve VII. (31)
The function of the buccal mucosa is a direct result of its structure. A tight spinosum layer and pump-functioning cells of the superficial layer provide protection from substances placed in the oral cavity. Elastin and collagen without bony attachment give the buccal mucosa flexibility and the ability to distend and compress. A rapid turnover rate and highly

vascularized lamina propria ensure quick healing after injury. The immune response is quickly aided by a lamina propria laden with lymphocytes and macrophages. (31)

The mucosa covering the lateral and under surface of the tongue is thin, smooth, and identical in structure with the lining of the rest of the oral cavity. Therefore it shares the same advantages such as easy harvesting, favorable immunologic properties (resistance to infection) and tissue characteristics (thick epithelium, high content of elastic fibers, thin lamina propria, rich vascularization) that are favorable properties for imbibition, inosculation, and revascularization of the graft. (27)

3. Harvesting the oral mucosa

Buccal mucosa may be harvested from the inner surface of the cheek or the inner surface of the upper or lower lip. For a single strip of buccal mucosa to be used as an onlay patch, the adult cheek provides up to 6 cm and the lip 4 cm length with 12 to 15 mm width. It is not advisable to continue the strip of buccal mucosa through the angle of the mouth to combine both cheek and lip segments in continuity for 10 cm. In the experience of Ransley, 1999 (12) the only buccal mucosa donor graft site complicated by a significant contracture was at the angle of the mouth. (12)

The mucosa of the cheek is preferable than that of the lip because the mucosa of the cheek is thicker and more robust than the mucosa of the lip. Also, the width of the lip limits the size of the graft. However in terms of outcomes, there is probably little difference between cheek and lip. (12)

General anesthesia via endotracheal intubation is the preferred method of airway control to facilitate access to the oral cavity. A surgical marking pen is used to outline the extent and shape of the graft away from the parotid papilla. The area should not encroach on the mental nerve, nor extend further back than the pterygomandibular raphe, and leave a cuff of mucosa 1 cm from the labial commissure. (14) The graft is better outlined as an elliptical shape, which eases closure of the anterior and posterior aspects of the donor site without compromising graft size or viability. A graft that is at least 10% longer and 10 - 20% wider than actually necessary is obtained to allow for shrinkage. (33)

Hydro-dissection of the oral mucosa from the underlying soft tissues using 1% lidocaine with 1:100,000 epinephrine and the the use of a No. 15 blade is recommended so that the incision is limited to the full thickness of the mucosa only. (34) Dissection of the buccinator muscle can lead to damage of the buccal neurovascular bundle. Also, branches of the facial nerve lying deep within this muscle would not be damaged by this incision. (9)

Harvesting the graft is slightly painful but not disabling in the post-operative period. Pain appears to be worse in the immediate post-operative period after suturing the harvest site. There is no difference in long-term post-operative morbidity whether the graft site is closed or left open however, some authors recommended to leave the buccal mucosa harvest sites unsutured. (35) Post-operative discomfort can be lessened by a diet of soft meals and by cleansing of the wound daily with povidone iodine solution. Some difficulty with mouth opening might be experienced during the early postoperative period but it will return to the normal range even if complications of wound healing have occurred. (9)

Harvesting lingual mucosal grafts follows the basic principles as that of the buccal mucosa with few differences. Harvesting the tongue should be technically easier than from the inner cheek since the tongue can be pulled out of the mouth with a traction suture. (Fig. 1)

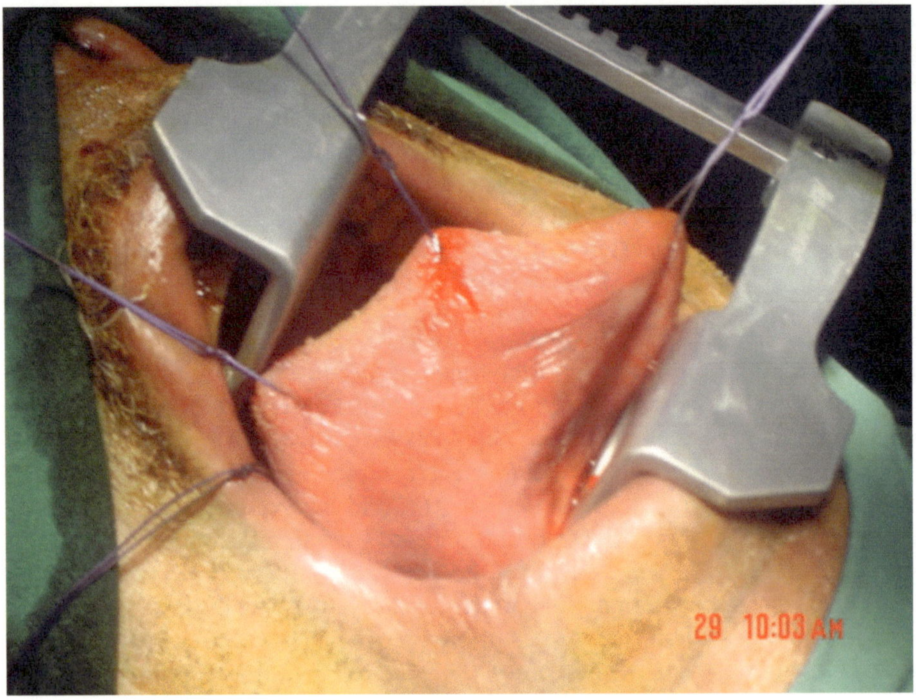

Fig. 1. Site of graft excision from lateral and undersurface of the tongue

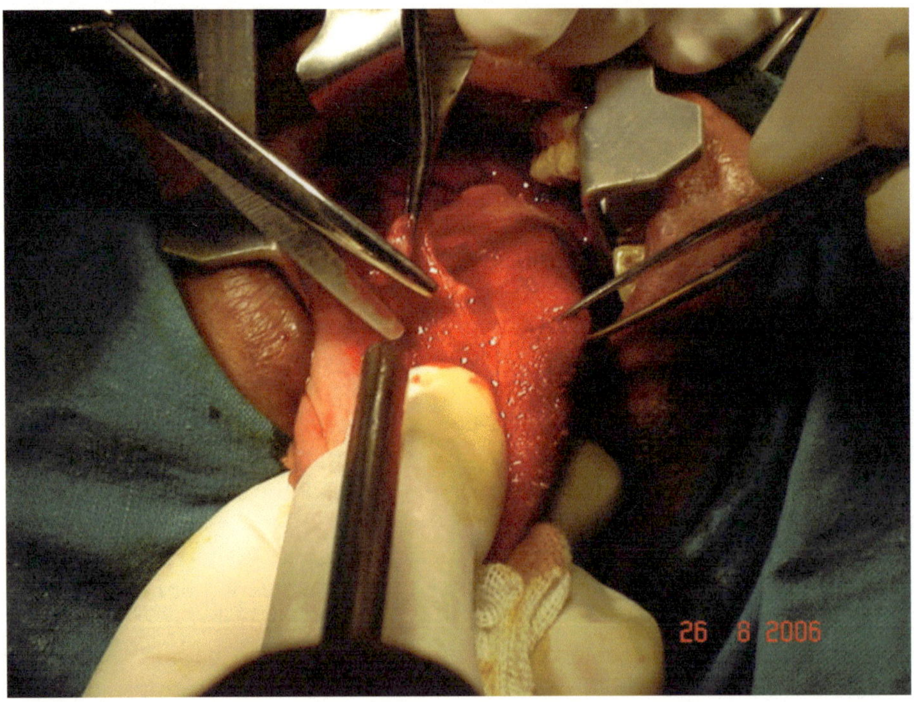

Fig. 2. Harvesting the graft

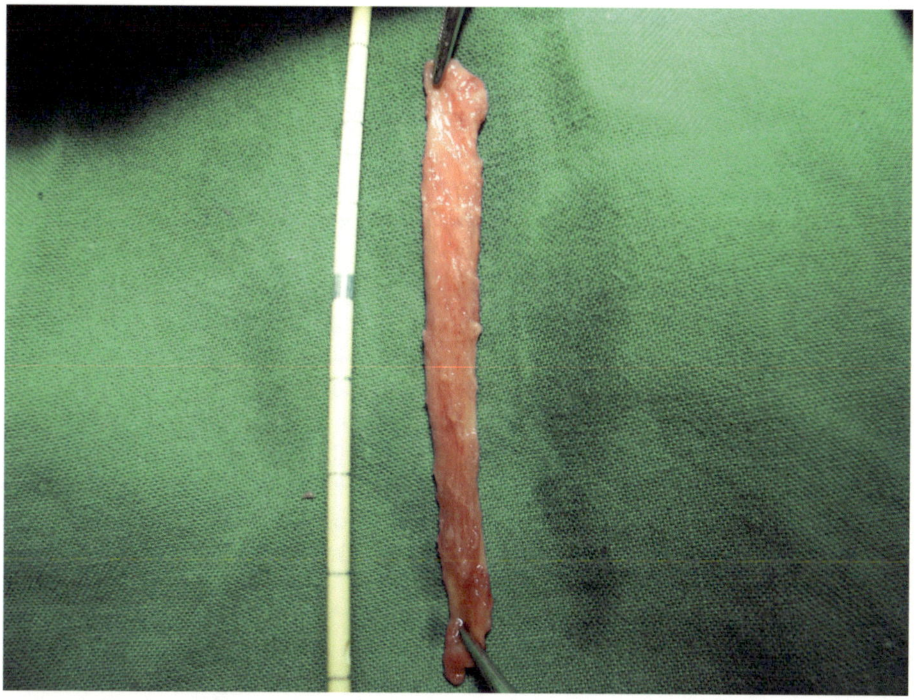

Fig. 3. Lingual graft excised

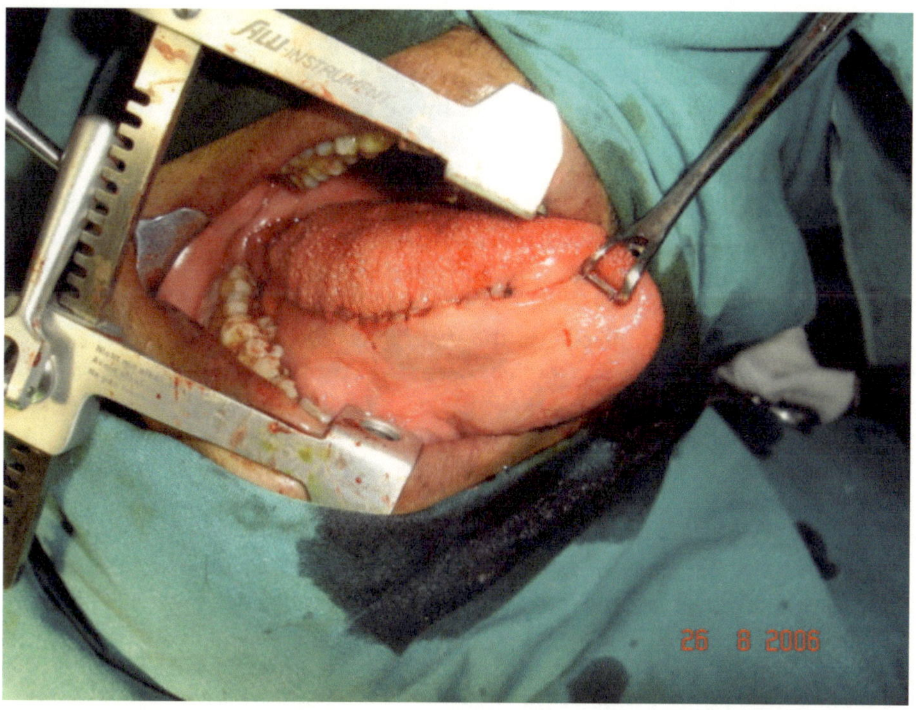

Fig. 4. Donor site closed

However, there is more bleeding associated with the lingual graft because the tongue is more vascular than the cheek. (25) During graft harvesting, care should be taken to the site of the opening of Wharton's duct and the underlying lingual nerve.

Simonato et al. (20) reported the lateral mucosal lining of the tongue as the harvest graft site since it is identical to the lining of the rest of the oral cavity and has no particular functional features. (20) Barbagli et al. (25) similarly described graft harvesting from the ventral surface of the tongue, suggesting that, when necessary, two grafts can be harvested from the same ventral tongue site. (25) In our description of the technique we suggested taking the graft from the lateral and undersurface of the tongue between the papillae situated on the dorsum and the sublingual mucosa. (29) (Fig. 2) Simonato, later admitted that the description of the surgical technique was inaccurate in his first report (36) and made clear that the site of the harvest graft is the ventrolateral mucosal surface of the tongue. (36)

In Barbagli's experience, the length of the lingual grafts was 4–6 cm (mean: 4.5 cm) with a width of 2.5 cm. (25) In our study, the length of the LMG used ranged from 4-10 cm and a width of 1.5 cm. (Fig. 3) Recently, Kumar et al. (26) reported harvesting a long (16.4 cm) and narrow (1–1.5 cm) lingual graft from the entire lateral mucosal lining of the tongue. (26)

In contrast to buccal mucosa the donor site must be closed with 4–0 polyglactin sutures at the end of the harvesting technique. (29) (Fig. 4)

4. Tips and tricks in the urethroplasty

Oral mucosa may be used as an onlay patch if the urethral plate is retained, as a complete tube if there is no available urethral plate or in various ways combined with other tissues. (30)

However, two main problems are faced using buccal mucosa as a tube graft. First, strips of oral mucosa should not be tubularized lengthwise to create 6 cm or 4cm tubes, because the width is insufficient. They can be folded lengthwise to provide shorter tubes of up to 3cm and 2cm, respectively or a second graft of similar dimensions can be applied to create a full-length cylinder of adequate diameter. (12)

Another problem with tube grafts in general is the inadequate graft take, as they are not circumferentially surrounded by vascularized tissue leading to increased incidence of contraction and anastomotic stricture that have led some to avoid tube grafts in favor of onlay procedure. (13, 37)

Traditionally, grafts have been placed on the ventral aspect of the urethra because it allows for easier access to the urethra and better visualization of the stricture. However, with a higher reported incidence of diverticula formation, due to poor support, and consequently postvoid dribbling and ejaculatory dysfunction. (38) Barbagli et al (39) introduced the dorsally placed graft and postulated that dorsal placement is advantageous as it allows better mechanical support for the graft with a richer vascular bed from the underlying corporeal bodies. (39) However, they recently compared the results of buccal mucosal urethroplasty in 50 patients with bulbar urethral strictures. Buccal mucosa grafts were placed on the ventral, dorsal and lateral bulbar urethral surface in 17, 27 and 6 cases, respectively. They reported that the placement of buccal mucosa grafts into the ventral, dorsal or lateral surface of the bulbar urethra showed the same success rates (83% to 85%) and the outcome was not affected by the surgical technique. Moreover, stricture recurrence was uniformly distributed in all patients. (40)

5. The process of take

The free graft initially adheres to its new bed by fibrin, and revascularization is achieved by the outgrowth of capillary buds from the recipient area to unite with those on the deep surface of the graft. This link up is usually well advanced by the third day. During this period (first 48 h.), the graft depends on imbibitions from the surrounding tissue. At the same time with the vascular link-up, the fibrin is infiltrated by fibroblasts, which gradually convert the initial weak adhesion provided by the fibrin clot into a definitive attachment by fibrous tissue. The strength of this attachment increases quickly, providing an anchorage within 4 days, which allows the graft to be handled safely if reasonable care is taken. More slowly a lymphatic link up is added and, even more slowly, nerve supply is re-established, although imperfectly and invariably. Of these various processes the ones most relevant in clinical practice are vascularization and fibrous tissue fixation. The speed with which this is accomplished, is determined by the characters of the bed on which the graft is laid, the characteristics of the graft itself, and the condition under which the graft is applied. (41)

The bed on which the graft is laid must have fibrinogen and the enzymes, which convert it into fibrin in sufficient quantities to provide the necessary adhesion. Sometimes the surface is harboring streptococcus pyogens, which destroys fibrin by its potent fibrinolysin action. Also, the bed should have enough blood supply to vascularize the graft. Rapid vascularization is important, and the distance to be traveled by the capillary buds in order to link-up clearly needs to be as short as possible. The graft has therefore to be in the closet possible contact with the bed. The most frequent cause of separation is bleeding from the bed; the resulting haematoma acts as a block to link-up of the outgrowing capillaries. (42)

The graft has also to lie immobile on the bed until it is firmly attached. In particular, shearing strains, which tend to make the graft slide to and fro and prevent capillary link-up, are to be avoided until the initial fibrin adhesion has been converted into a strong fibrous tissue anchorage. (42)

In summary, the graft take requires a bed that is capable of providing the necessary capillary outgrowth to vascularize a graft, free of pathogens inimical to graft take in addition to an immobile close contact between graft and bed. The most frequent cause of graft loss is the presence of a hematoma which separates the graft from its bed and or shearing movements which prevent adhesion between graft and bed, each in its own way preventing capillary link up and vascularization. (42)

6. Indications

In patients with congenital or acquired urethral defects, short or lengthy segments of the urethra need to be reconstructed. Vascularized preputial and penile shaft skin flaps are frequently used to achieve this. (43)

After repeated previous surgery there is lacking of penile and preputial skin and the blood supply of these skin flaps is disturbed so that free graft material is preferred. Free skin graft material from extragenital regions is less suitable due to the thickness, hair growth or tendency to contract. The use of bladder mucosal free graft includes the additional and not inconsiderable burden for the patient arising from graft harvesting, and is procedurally quite complicated. Furthermore, postoperative complications caused by cauliflower-like deformities in the meatus externus urethrae are frequent. These aspects have greatly reduced the potential of this operating technique. (5)

The first very good results of buccal mucosa as a free graft encourage its usage in these situations. El-Kassaby and associates, 1993 (11) recommended the use of buccal mucosal graft in the treatment of anterior urethral stricture. They used this technique for treatment of short strictures (1 to 2cm) that usually required a 2 to 4 cm repair, making excision and end-to-end anastomosis impractical. Buccal mucosa has also been used to replace urethra in epispadias repairs in exstrophy patients whose penile skin is insufficient. (44)
So, we can summarize the current indications for the use of buccal mucosal free grafts for substitution urethroplasty in:

- Anterior urethral strictures.
- Proximal hypospadias especially in circumcised patients.
- Crippled hypospadias where there is no sufficient genital skin.
- Epispadias when the penile skin is insufficient.

7. Advantages

- Easily accessible, non-hair bearing and the supply source is constant and adequate.
- The intraoral donor site guarantees an excellent cosmetic result.
- The graft is extremely elastic and shows only a slight tendency to contraction.
- The graft has been noted to retain the elasticity of the virgin tissue.
- The meatal problems of excoriation, encrustation and protuberance that encountered with bladder mucosa, have not been a problem with buccal mucosa.
- High resistance to infection and trauma and high regenerative power.
- Buccal mucosa is characterized by thick epithelial layer and thin lamina propria that make the graft mechanically stiff and easy handled and aid in rapid vascularization of the graft.

8. Disadvantages

- The oral mucosa cannot be tubularized to create long tubes because the width is insufficient. So, it can be folded lengthwise to provide shorter tubes or a second flap of similar dimensions can be applied to create a full-length cylinder of adequate diameter.
- It may lead to a significant contracture at the angle of the mouth if the buccal mucosal graft is taken through the angle.
- Liability of injury to superficial branches of the facial nerve.
- Stricture and fistula continue to be a problem with buccal mucosa as with any other free graft.

9. Results of oral mucosa urethroplasty

There is no doubt, both subjectively and objectively, that oral mucosa is proving very satisfactory as a material for urethral reconstruction. This may be due to growth factors within the mucosa that promote rapid healing, revascularization occurs quickly because of the thin lamina propria and the originally highly vascular bed from which the buccal mucosal graft was taken. (43)
In their early report of the use of buccal mucosa in hypospadias repair, Dessanti and associates, 1992 (10) reported only one case of urethral fistula out of 8 hypospadias patients

after 6-18 months of follow up. Another two patients required urethral dilatation during the initial 4 weeks because of mild anastomotic stenosis. No meatal problems such as stenosis or granulomatous reactions was observed. (10)

Similarly, Burger and associates (9) in the same year used buccal mucosa in 6 patients; failed hypospadias repair (3), severe stricture after hypospadias repair (1), short urethra (1) and epispadias in 1 patient. The results were 3 urethral fistulae and 1 meatal stenosis in 3 patients. No urethral stricture or diverticulum was noted, and the final outcome was good functionally and cosmetically in all patients. (9)

One year later El-Kasaby and associates (11) reported their experience with buccal mucosa patch graft in the management of 20 patients with anterior urethral strictures. Results were excellent in 18 patients while 2 required revision for recurrent stricture. (11)

The experience of Ransley and Manzoni, 1999 (12) with buccal mucosal graft extended to more than a 100 case. They reported a secondary operation rate of approximately 20%, which are mostly due to minor fistulae or the need for meatal revision. Radical reoperation with further urethral augmentation with an additional buccal mucosal graft had been necessary on some occasions. They recommended the use of preoperative testosterone treatment in difficult cases to improve the vascularity of the penile skin and thereby enhance the chances of success with a free graft technique. (12)

Barbagli and associates (39) have an extensive experience in the use of buccal mucosa for treatment of anterior urethral strictures. In 1998, they reported the use of buccal mucosa as a dorsal onlay graft in the management of 6 adult patients with bulbourethral strictures. The results were excellent with no stricture recurred in 6 patients. (39) In 2007, (45) they reported the results of 94 patients who underwent bulbar urethral reconstruction using two dorsal onlay techniques, namely augmented anastomotic urethroplasty and dorsal onlay graft urethroplasty. Forty-eight out of 94 patients received skin grafts and 46 buccal mucosal grafts. Twenty-eight (58.3%) out of 48 penile skin grafts were successful and 20 (41.7%) failed. Thirty-six (78.3%) out of 46 buccal mucosa grafts were successful and 10 (21.7%) failed. They concluded that buccal mucosa seems to be the best substitute graft material for bulbar urethroplasty using dorsal approach. (45)

More recently, Palminteri and associates, 2008 (15) used buccal mucosa as combined dorsal plus ventral graft in 48 patients with bulbar urethral stricture where 43(89.6%) patients were successful and 5(10.4%) patients showed failures in the form of recurrence of the stricture. (15)

In 2002, we reported our results of the use of three different types of free grafts (skin, bladder and buccal) in urethral reconstruction. The results showed that buccal mucosal graft had the highest success rate. Buccal mucosal graft was used in 25 patients, 10 hypospadias and 15 patients with urethral stricture. As regard the hypospadias patients (40%) were primary and (60%) were redo cases. The buccal mucosa was applied as patch graft in all patients. The length of the grafts ranged from 2.5-6 cm. The success rate was (70%) where 3 patients showed 4 complications in the form of 2 fistulae, one meatal stenosis and one breakdown. In urethral stricture patients, (26.7%) were primary and (73.3%) were secondary cases. The stricture was bulbar in all patients. The buccal mucosal graft was applied as patch graft in all patients. The length of the graft ranged from 3-5cm. Four patients showed 4 complications in the form of one urethrocutaneous fistula, one neourethral stenosis and 2 anastomotic strictures. The fistula was minute and closed spontaneously. The final success rate was (80%). (46)

At that time, we concluded that urethral reconstruction using buccal mucosa is a useful technique and the results appear to be acceptable given the difficulty of the cases in which buccal mucosa was used. The structure, function and ease of working with buccal mucosa make it the ideal extragenital source for reconstruction of the urethra in complex hypospadias and urethral stricture. Easiness of harvesting and rapid healing process also contributes to its superiority. As in all urethral reconstructions, the learning curve is long. However, as one becomes more familiar with urethral reconstruction using buccal mucosa, no doubt the complication rate will decrease measurably. (46)

Among the good results of the oral mucosa urethroplasty, the lingual mucosa is no exception. In their pioneering report, Simonato et al (20) reported seven successful cases out of the 8 cases included in his study achieving a success rate of 87.5%. (20) In a following report, they reported a series of 29 patients with anterior urethral strictures who underwent urethral reconstruction using LMG. The mean stricture length was 3.6 cm (range, 1.5–9.0 cm). The length of the LMG used ranged from 3 cm to 9 cm (mean, 5.3 cm), with a mean width of 1.5 cm. Mean follow-up time was 17.7 months (range, 6–71 months). The overall early stricture recurrence was 20.7%. (27)

Since then a number of groups have investigated the feasibility of lingual mucosa graft urethroplasty (16, 17, 21-23, 25, 26, 29, 30, 36, 47) whether experimentally (17, 21) or clinically, (16, 22, 23, 25, 26, 29, 30, 36, 47) alone or with buccal mucosa, (16, 17) and with different urethroplasty techniques. (23, 26, 47)

Barbagli et al (25) later described their early experience using LMG for urethral reconstruction in 10 patients with anterior urethral strictures. The length of urethral strictures was 2–6 cm and the length of the lingual grafts was 4–6 cm (mean, 4.5 cm) with a width of 2.5 cm. Mean follow-up time was 5 months (range, 3–12 months); nine cases (90%) were successful. (25)

We have also described our early results of lingual mucosa urethroplasty in 18 patients with long recurrent strictures of the anterior urethra. (29) Their mean age was 39.5 years (18-66 years), and the mean stricture length was 4.36 cm (3-9 cm). Of the 18 cases, 6 were penile, 8 bulbar, and 4 bulbopenile. The primary etiology was traumatic in 8 cases, iatrogenic in 6 cases, and inflammatory in 4 cases. Previous stricture treatments included dilations in all 18 patients, optical internal urethrotomy in 14, hypospadias repair in 2, and failed BMG urethroplasty in 2. The graft was placed dorsally in 12 cases and ventrally in 6 cases. The mean operative time was about 177 mins (140-210 mins) using a one-team approach. The length of the LMG used ranged from 4-10 cm and a width of 1.5 cm. The graft was harvested unilaterally in 15 (83%) cases and bilaterally in 3 (17%) cases. There was no need for intraoperative blood transfusions, and there were no major perioperative complications. (29)

There were 15 successful cases (83.3%), 2 patients had restricture at the anastomotic site, and 1 patient showed a urethrocutaneous fistula. In the successful cases, there were no residual strictures and no urethral diverticulae or sacculations in their urethrograms at 3 months. The peak flow rate improved from a mean of 4.98 ml/s (0.6-8.6 ml/s) to 27.28 ml/s (22.4-39.6 ml/s). Urethroscopy was done in 10 out of the 15 successful cases and revealed that LMGs were almost indistinguishable from the native urethra. (29)

In another prospective randomized controlled study, we compared outcomes as well as donor site complications of buccal mucosal graft (BMG) (20 patients) versus lingual mucosal graft (LMG) (20 patients) dorsal onlay urethroplasty in 40 patients with anterior urethral

strictures. Early and late complications, success rate and patient satisfaction were compared between the two groups.
The number of patients with pendulous, bulbar and bulbopendulous strictures as well as the mean stricture length and mean follow-up were comparable between the two groups. No significant difference between both groups in the operative time, hospital stay, early postoperative pain and time to resume fluid intake and normal diet. Late after surgery, the postoperative pain, perioral numbness and tightness of the mouth as well as changes in salivary function were significantly higher in the buccal mucosa (BMG) group versus the lingual mucosa (LMG) group ($p < 0.01$). The success rate in both groups was similar (90% in the BMG group and 85% in the LMG group) ($p > 0.05$). In the BMG group 80% and in the LMG group 85% said they would recommend this procedure to another patient ($p > 0.05$). (16)
Recently, Xu et al (47) published the biggest lingual mucosa urethroplasty series in 92 cases. After a mean follow-up of 17.2 months, complications reported in 8 patients, including urinary fistulas in 4 patients; recurrent strictures developed in 4 patients at 3–4 months post-operatively. (47)

10. Conclusion

Being easy to harvest and to handle, immune to infections and accustomed to a wet enviroment, the oral mucosa displays many inherent characteristics of an ideal graft substitute for urethroplasty.

11. References

[1] Duckett JW. Transverse preputial island flap technique for repair of severe hypospadias. Urol Clin North Am. 1980;7:423-430.

[2] Mitchell ME, Adams MC, Rink RC. Urethral replacement with ureter. J Urol. 1988;139:1282-1285.

[3] Snow BW, Cartwright PC. Tunica vaginalis urethroplasty. Urology. 1992;40:442-445.

[4] Hendren WH, Crooks KK. Tubed free skin graft for construction of male urethra. J Urol. 1980;123:858-861.

[5] Ehrlich RM, Reda EF, Koyle MA, Kogan SJ, Levitt SB. Complications of bladder mucosal graft. J Urol. 1989;142:626-627.

[6] Filipas D, Wahlmann U, Hohenfellner R. History of oral mucosa. Eur Urol. 1998;34:165-168.

[7] Humby G, Higgins TT. A one stage operation for hypospadias. British Journal of Surgery. 1941;29:84-92.

[8] editor. 1986; Southhampton, England: 1986.

[9] Burger RA, Muller SC, el-Damanhoury H, Tschakaloff A, Riedmiller H, Hohenfellner R. The buccal mucosal graft for urethral reconstruction: a preliminary report. J Urol. 1992;147:662-664.

[10] Dessanti A, Rigamonti W, Merulla V, Falchetti D, Caccia G. Autologous buccal mucosa graft for hypospadias repair: an initial report. J Urol. 1992; 147:1081-1083.

[11] el-Kasaby AW, Fath-Alla M, Noweir AM, el-Halaby MR, Zakaria W, el-Beialy MH. The use of buccal mucosa patch graft in the management of anterior urethral strictures. J Urol. 1993;149:276.

[12] Ransley PG, Manzoni GM. Buccal mucosa graft for hypospadias. In: Ehrlich RE, Alter GJ, editors. Reconstructive and Plastic Surgery of the external Genitalia, Adult and Pediatric. Philadelphia, PA: WB Saunders company; 1999. p. 121.

[13] Bhargava S, Chapple CR. Buccal mucosal urethroplasty: Is it the new gold standard? BJU Int. 2004;93:1191-1193.

[14] Fabbroni G, Loukota RA, Eardley I. Buccal mucosal grafts for urethroplasty: Surgical technique and morbidity. Br J Oral Maxillofac Surg. 2005;43:320-323.

[15] Palminteri E, Manzoni G, Berdondini E et al. Combined dorsal plus ventral double buccal mucosa graft in bulbar urethral reconstruction. Eur Urol. 2008;53:81-89.

[16] Elgamal S, Ragab MM, Farahat Y, Elnady M, Elsharaby M, Abo Farha O. A prospective randomized study comparing buccal and lingual mucosal dorsal onlay graft for management of anterior urehral strictures. Tanta Medical Journal. 2008;36:597-608.

[17] Hu X, Xu Y, Song L, Zhang H. Combined Buccal and Lingual Mucosa Grafts for Urethroplasty: An Experimental Study in Dogs. J Surg Res. 2009

[18] Kumar A, Das SK, Trivedi S, Dwivedi US, Singh PB. Substitution urethroplasty for anterior urethral strictures: buccal versus lingual mucosal graft. Urol Int. 2010;84:78-83.

[19] Singh O, Gupta SS, Arvind NK. Anterior urethral strictures: a brief review of the current surgical treatment. Urol Int. 2011;86:1-10.

[20] Simonato A, Gregori A, Lissiani A et al. The tongue as an alternative donor site for graft urethroplasty: a pilot study. J Urol. 2006;175:589-592.

[21] Song LJ, Xu YM, Hu XY, Zhang HZ. Urethral substitution using autologous lingual mucosal grafts: an experimental study. BJU Int. 2008;101:739-743.

[22] Simonato A, Gregori A. Oral complications after lingual mucosal graft harvest for urethroplasty. ANZ J Surg. 2008;78:933-934.

[23] Singh PB, Das SK, Kumar A et al. Dorsal onlay lingual mucosal graft urethroplasty: Comparison of two techniques. Int J Urol. 2008;15:1002-1005.

[24] Trivedi S, Kumar A, Goyal NK, Dwivedi US, Singh PB. Urethral reconstruction in balanitis xerotica obliterans. Urol Int. 2008;81:285-289.

[25] Barbagli G, De Angelis M, Romano G, Ciabatti PG, Lazzeri M. The use of lingual mucosal graft in adult anterior urethroplasty: Surgical steps and short-term outcome. Eur Urol. 2008;54:671-676.

[26] Kumar A, Das SK, Sharma GK et al. Lingual mucosal graft substitution urethroplasty for anterior urethral strictures: our technique of graft harvesting. World J Urol. 2008;26:275-280.

[27] Simonato A, Gregori A, Ambruosi C et al. Lingual mucosal graft urethroplasty for anterior urethral reconstruction. Eur Urol. 2008;54:79-85.

[28] Das SK, Kumar A, Sharma GK et al. Lingual mucosal graft urethroplasty for anterior urethral strictures. Urology. 2009;73:105-108.

[29] Ragab MM, Elgamal S, Farahat Y, Saber W, Hawas M, Elsharaby M. Urethroplasty with lingual mucosal graft for management of long and recurrent strictures of the anterior urethra. Urotoday Int J. 2009;2

[30] Xu YM, Sa YL, Fu Q, Zhang J, Si JM, Liu ZS. Oral mucosal grafts urethroplasty for the treatment of long segmented anterior urethral strictures. World J Urol. 2009;27:565-571.

[31] Brock JW, Nelson E. Buccal mucosa reconstruction of the urethra. In: Ehrlich RE, Alter GJ, editors. Reconstructive and Plastic Surgery of the External Genitalia, Adult and Pediatric. WB Saunders company; 1999. p. 126.

[32] Strachan DS, Avery JK. Histology of the oral mucosa and tonsils. In: Avery JK, editor. Oral development and histology. Thieme Medical Publishers; 2001. p. 243.

[33] Wood DN, Allen SE, Andrich DE, Greenwell TJ, Mundy AR. The morbidity of buccal mucosa graft harvest for urethroplasty and the effect of nonclosure of the graft harvest site on postoperative pain. J Urol. 2004;172:580-583.

[34] Markiewicz MR, Margarone JE, Barbagli G, Scannapieco FA. Oral mucosa harvest: An overview of anatomic and biologic considerations. EAU-EBU update series. 2007;5:179-187.

[35] Muruganandam K, Dubey D, Gulia AK et al. Closure versus nonclosure of buccal mucosal graft harvest site: A prospective randomized study on postoperative morbidity. Indian J Urol. 2009;25:72-75.

[36] Simonato A, Gregori A. Lingual mucosal grafts for anterior urethroplasty: a review. BJU Int. 2010;105:132-133.

[37] Woodall JR, Gosalbez R, Barone J, Perez LM. Buccal mucosa: Free grafts in complicated urethral reconstruction. Reconstructive Surgery of the Lower Urinary Tract in Children. Oxford: Isis Medical Media; 1995. p. 29.

[38] Wessels H, McAninch JW. Use of free grafts in urethral stricture reconstruction. J Urol. 1996;155:1912-1915.

[39] Barbagli G, Palminteri E, Rizzo M. Dorsal onlay graft urethroplasty using penile skin or buccal mucosa in adult bulbourethral strictures. J Urol. 1998;160:1307-1309.

[40] Barbagli G, Palminteri E, Guazzoni G, Montorsi F, Turini D, Lazzeri M. Bulbar urethroplasty using buccal mucosa grafts placed in the ventral, dorsal or lateral surface of the urethra: Are results affected by the surgical technique? J Urol. 2005;174:955-958.

[41] Triana RJJ, Murakami CS, Larrabee WFJ. Skin grafts and local flaps. In: Papel ID, editor. Facial Plastic and Reconstructive Surgery. New York, NY: Thieme Medical Publishers; 2009. p. 41.

[42] McGregor AD, McGregor IA. Free Skin Grafts. In: McGregor AD, McGregor IA, editors. Fundamental Techniques of Plastic Surgery and their Surgical Applications. Philadelphia, Pa,: Churchill Livingstone; 2000. p. 35-59.

[43] Duckett JW, Coplen D, Ewalt D, Baskin LS. Buccal mucosal urethral replacement. J Urol. 1995;153:1660-1663.

[44] Dessanti A, Iannuccelli M, Ginesu G, Feo C. Reconstruction of hypospadias and epispadias with buccal mucosa free graft as primary surgery: more than 10 years of experience. J Urol. 2003;170:1600.

[45] Barbagli G, Lazzeri M. History and evolution of dorsal onlay urethroplasty for bulbar urethral stricture repair using skin or buccal mucosal grafts. Urologia. 2007;74:233.
[46] Haroun H. Evaluation of three different free grafts in urethral reconstruction. [dissertation]. Tanta, Egypt: M.D Thesis in Urology,Tanta University; 2002.
[47] Xu YM, Fu Q, Sa YL et al. Treatment of urethral strictures using lingual mucosas urethroplasty: experience of 92 cases. Chin Med J (Engl). 2010;123:458-462.

9

Mechanism of Penile Prosthesis Induced Urethral Stricture: Treatment and Prevention

Jong Kwan Park and Chen Zhao
Chonbuk National University
South Korea

1. Introduction

The advent of phosphodiesterase type 5 inhibitor has revolutionized the management of erectile dysfunction (ED). Since the introduction of sildenafil citrate in 1998, oral systemic therapy has become the first line therapy for men with ED. However, oral pharmacotherapy often fails in patients with severe diabetes, radical prostatectomy, Peyronie's disease, and severe penile fibrosis. These patients may select other therapies such as penile injection therapy or a vacuum erection device. When oral and injectable therapies fail to produce satisfactory results, implantation of a penile prosthesis is the last strategy which has demonstrated the highest level of satisfaction among treatments for ED [1,2].

Penile implants include malleable (semi-rigid) and inflatable (two- or three-piece) types. Most patients prefer the three-piece inflatable devices because it most closely approaches the functioning penis with respect to flaccidity and erection. Three-piece prostheses consist of paired corporal cylinders, a scrotal pump, and a large volume reservoir implanted into the prevesical or retropubic space (Fig. 1). Currently available three-piece devices include the Coloplast Titan, Coloplast Titan Narrow Base, the AMS Ultrex, the AMS 700 CX, AMS 700 CXM and the AMS 700 CXR. A major difference is whether connecting tubing between cylinders and pump has been made on production line or not.

The inflatable prostheses are usually inserted via a penoscrotal or an infrapubic approach. The advantage of the infrapubic approach is the placement of the reservoir under direct vision. However, this approach limits to expose the corpora cavernosa and may damage the dorsal nerve, especially during revision procedures. The penoscrotal or transverse scrotal approach allows to securely placing the pump in the scrotum and the skin in the prepubic area is not violated, but the reservoir has to be placed blindly through the inguinal canal which may injury the iliac vessels [3].

In the past, the implantation of a penile prosthesis was often associated with high complication rate such as infection, persistent pain, cavernous perforation, mechanical failure, malposition, erosion into the bladder, urethra and bowel, and gangrene [4,5]. In recent years, the use of antibiotic impregnated or hydrophilic-coated prosthesis and proper antibiotic prophylaxis against Gram-positive and Gram-negative bacteria has significantly reduced the complication rates. The two main complications of penile prosthesis implantation are mechanical failures and infection. The technical improvements result in mechanical failure rates of less than 5% at 5-year follow-up [6,7], and infection rates range from 1 to 4% [8,9].

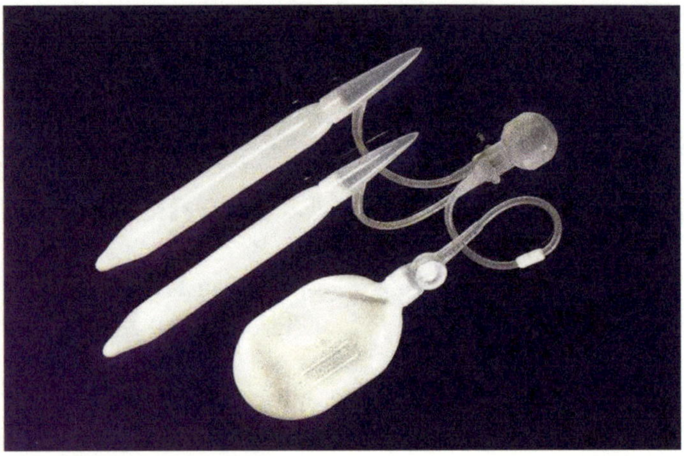

Fig. 1. Coloplast Titan inflatable penile prosthesis

Urethral stricture after implantation of a three-piece inflatable penile prosthesis is very rare but has been reported in 2007 [10]. Urethral stricture was induced by compression of twisted tubing in three-piece inflatable penile prosthesis and it would be aggravated with the lapse of time [11]. We developed a more reliable surgical technique to place the three-piece inflatable penile prosthesis. Also, we would like to share the unusual experience which may be helpful to prevent urethral stricture in penile prosthesis implantation.

2. Urethral stricture

The normal urethral spongiosum was comprised of 75.1% type I collagen and 24.9% type III collagen. A functional nerve supply to the urethral spongiosum seems to be crucial in the maintenance of the unique ultrastructure of the urethral spongiosum [12]. The term urethral stricture refers to urethral disease and is a scarring process of the subepithelial tissue of the corpus spongiosum that constricts the urethral lumen [13]. Recent studies on molecular mechanism of urethral stricture have shown that the fibrosis in strictures is different from other organ in the wound healing process. In the process of the urethral stricture, the type I collagen in urethral stricture tissue was significantly increased (83.9%), with a corresponding decrease in type III collagen (16.1%) [14]. The fibrotic process may also be associated with significant changes in nitric oxide synthase metabolism. The connective tissue growth factor was significantly up-regulated in urethral tissues of urethral stricture patients, which has been identified as a cause of other fibrotic diseases [15].

The etiology includes idiopathic, iatrogenic, inflammatory, and traumatic. In an evaluation of 175 patients, it showed that most urethral strictures are idiopathic (34%) or iatrogenic (32%), being less frequently inflammatory (20%) or traumatic (14%) [16]. Patients who have urethral strictures most often present with obstructive voiding symptoms or urinary tract infections such as prostatitis and epididymitis. Some patients also present with urinary retention [13].

2.1 Mechanism of urethral stricture by penile prosthesis

The paired corporal cylinders and scrotal pump of the three-piece prosthesis are connected by tubeings. If a cylinder were abnormally rotated 360 degree from neutral position during the implantation, the tubeing connected the cylinder would be rotated as well. The rotated tubeing compresses the urethra and induces inflammation in the corpus spongiosum which results in urethral stricture.

2.2 Diagnosis of urethral stricture

Urethral stricture could be diagnosed by urine analysis, voiding symptoms aggravated just after implantation, uroflowmetry and retrograde urethrography. Before or during surgery, endoscopy (Fig. 2) or bougienage (urethral sound) could be used to evaluate the stricture and ensure completely, all the involved urethra is included in the reconstruction.

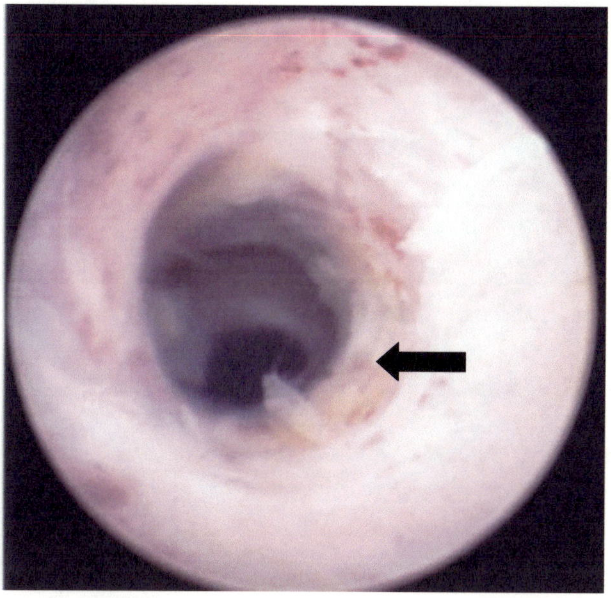

Fig. 2. Cystoscopy reveals penile urethral stricture (arrow) after three-piece penile prosthesis (Mentor alpha I) implantation 6 months later

2.3 Prevention and treatment

During the implantation, cylinder, tubing, and pump must be placed without abnormal rotation. If you find the rotated tubing or pump induced by the abnormal rotation of the cylinder, you have to relocate the cylinder after re-rotation of the abnormal rotated cylinder (Fig. 3).

3. Unusual experience of long urethral stricture by rotated tubeing

A 36-year-old man was presented with severe voiding difficulty after implantation of the three-piece inflatable penile prosthesis. The symptom occurred after removal of a Foley catheter at day 1 of implantation postoperatively and voiding difficulty continued. Previously, he had received an inflatable penile prosthesis Mentor Alpha I implantation (Mentor Corp., Santa Barbara, CA, USA) via infrapubic approach 4.5 years ago. We performed uroflowmetry and retrograde urethrography. The peak uroflowrate was 4 mL/second, and retrograde urethrogram showed severe penile urethral stricture (Fig. 4).

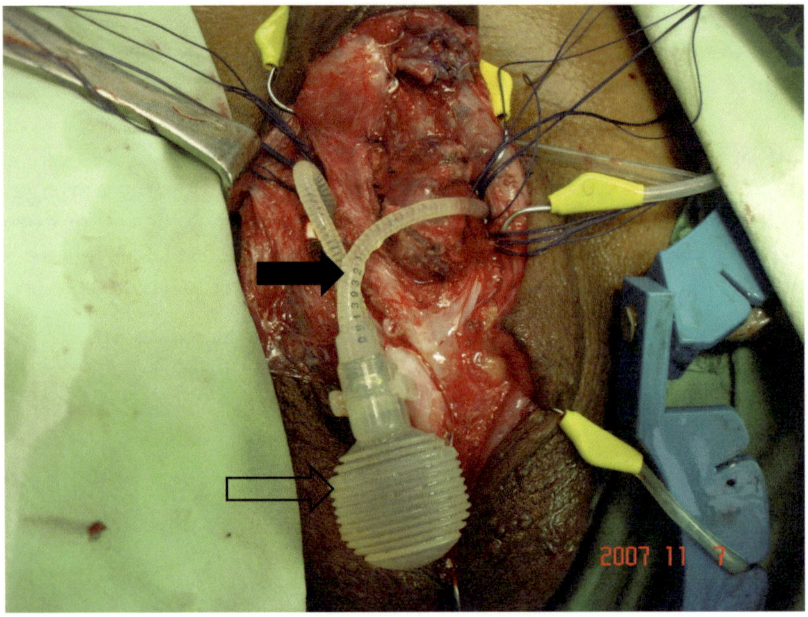

Fig. 3. Rotated tubeings (solid arrow) and pump (open arrow)

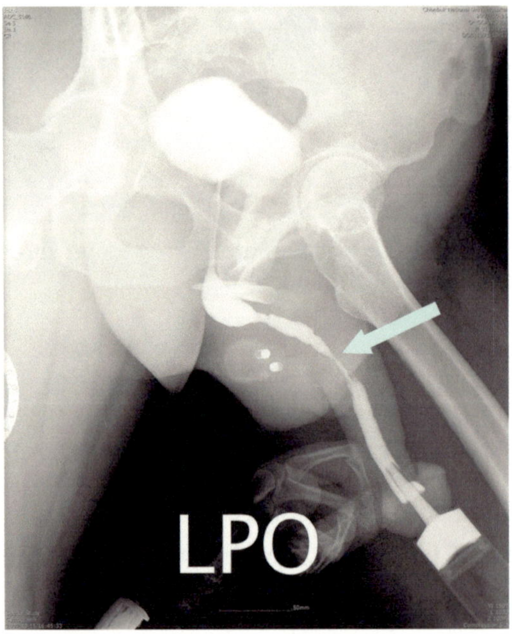

Fig. 4. Retrograde urethrogram shows severe urethral stricture (solid arrow)

During the revision surgery, we made a neourethra with pedicle island of penile skin and anastomosed after removal of the strictured portion (Fig. 5). After urethroplasty, new cylinders and pump were placed in cavernosal spaces and intra-scrotum in a routine manner, respectively (Fig. 6).

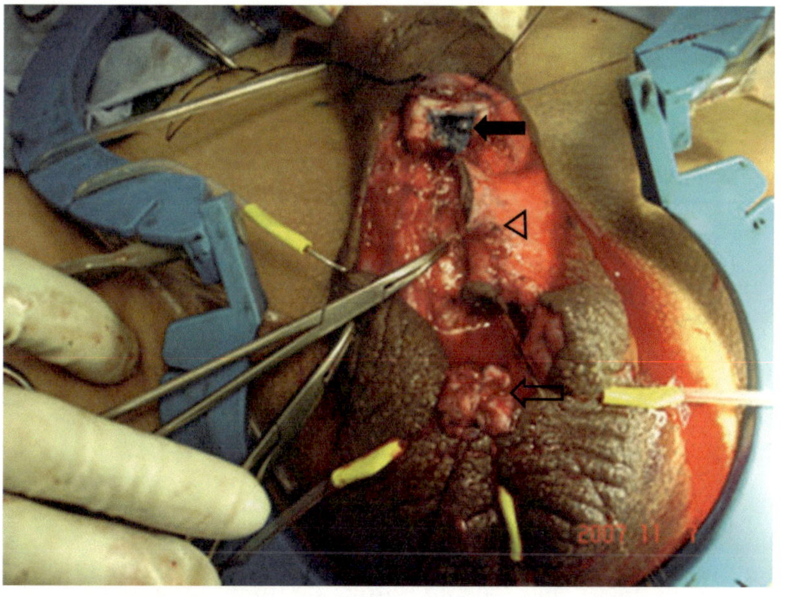

Fig. 5. Operative view shows long urethral defect between distal (solid arrow) and proximal (open arrow) urethral opening and neourethra with pedicle island of penile skin (open arrow head)

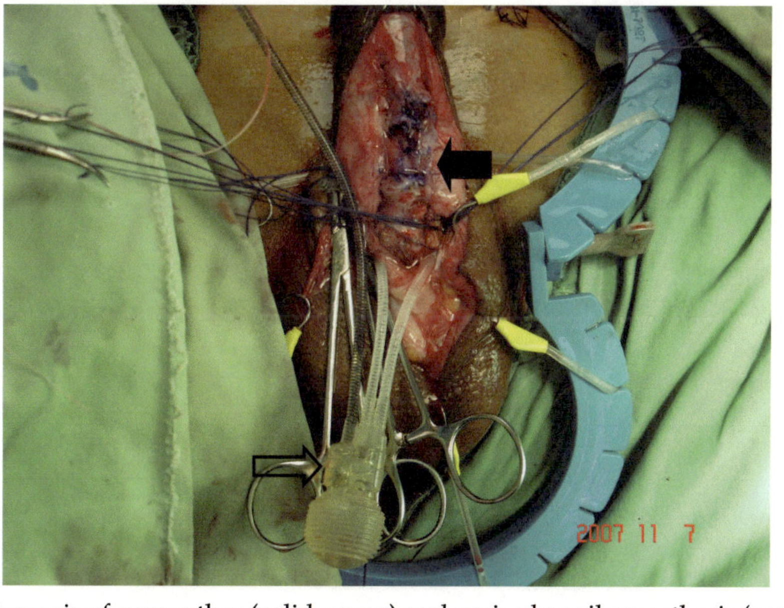

Fig. 6. Anastomosis of neourethra (solid arrow) and revised penile prosthesis (open arrow). Pump is located at the neutral position (open arrow)

We have drawn two longitudinal lines on the cylinder and tubings leading from cylinder to prevent the abnormal rotation of the cylinder during the preparation of the prosthesis (Fig. 7). If the cylinder would be rotated, a marked line at the related tubeing also is twisted.

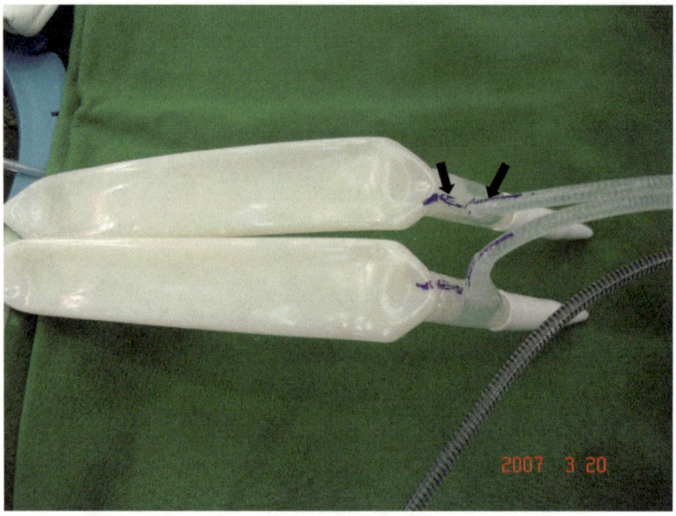

Fig. 7. Two longitudinal lines marked at the cylinder and tubeings

We removed a Foley catheter and took an retrograde urethrography on postoperative day 21. However, there was dye extravasation from the anastomosed portion to the pump (Fig. 8).

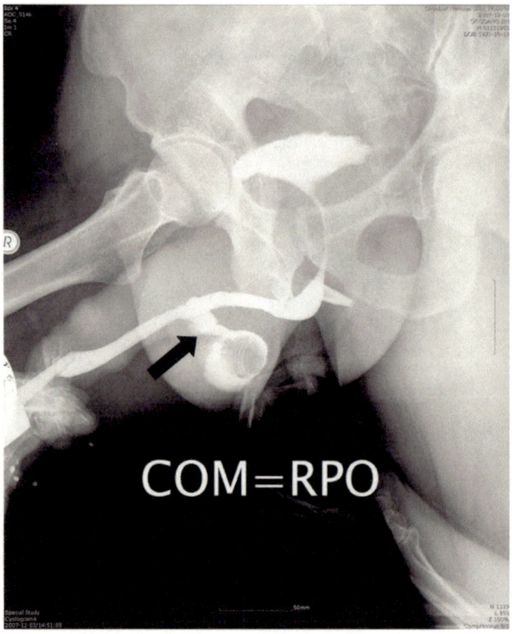

Fig. 8. Retrograde urethrogram shows the extravastion of dye from the anastomotic portion to the pump (solid arrow)

A 16 Fr Foley catheter was inserted again, and prescribed oral antibiotics for additional 21 days. We performed voiding cystourethrography at day 21 after the second insertion of a Foley catheter. There was no extravasation in the urethra (Fig. 9).

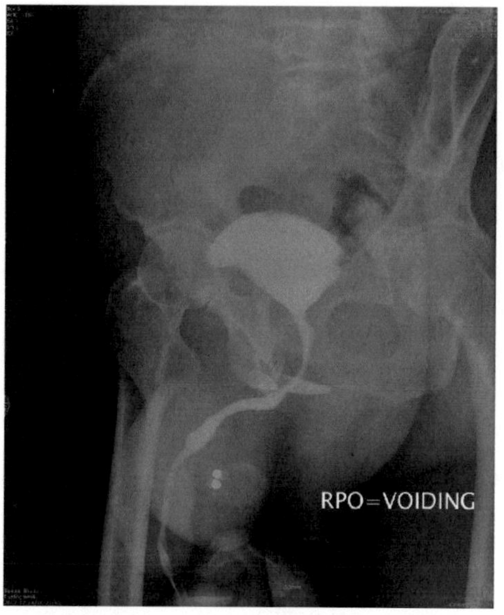

Fig. 9. Voiding cystogram do not shows extravasation of dye

4. Conclusions

During the implantation of a three piece inflatable penile prosthesis, abnormal rotation of the cylinder rotates the connecting tubeing between cylinder and pump. If the operator ignores the abnormal rotated cylinder, the rotated tubeing compress the urethra resulting in urethral stricture. The stricture induced by compression by the rotated tubeing will be aggravated with the duration of the time. We suggest the following surgical tips to prevent urethral stricture in penile implantation of a three-piece of penile prosthesis, which was produced company of Coloplast. (i) An incision of the tunica albuginea may be made as laterally as possible to prevent tubing crossing the anterior urethra. (ii) The producer or operator should mark two longitudinal lines parallel to the long axis of the cylinder at the surface of the cylinders and tubings leading from the cylinders during the preparation of penile prosthesis. (iii) Stitches are to be made on the scrotal soft tissue to prevent rotation of the pump. (iv) The pump should be placed at the lowest dependent portion.

5. Acknowledgment

This study was supported by grants of Clinical Trial Center Medical Device and Research Institute for Medical Sciences of Chonbuk National University Hospital and of the Korea Healthcare Technology R&D Project, Ministry for Health, Welfare &Family Affairs, Republic of Korea (A091220).

6. References

[1] Holloway, FB. & Farah, RN. (1997). Intermediate term assessment of the reliability, function and patient satisfaction with the AMS700 Ultrex penile prosthesis. *Journal of Urology* 157(5): 1687-1691.

[2] Tefilli, MV., Dubocq, F., Rajpurkar, A., Gheiler, EL., Tiguert, R., Barton, C., Li, H. & Dhabuwala, CB. (1998). Assessment of psychosexual adjustment after insertion of inflatable penile prosthesis. *Urology* 52(6): 1106-1112.

[3] Mulcahy, JJ., Austoni, E., Barada, JH., Choi, HK., Hellstrom, WJ., Krishnamurti, S., Moncada, I., Schultheiss, D., Sohn, M. & Wessells, H. (2004). The penile implant for erectile dysfunction. *Journal of Sexual Medicine* 1(1): 98-109.

[4] Wilson, Sk., Delk, JR., Mulcahy, JJ., Cleves, M. & Salem, E. (2006). Upsizing of inflatable penile implant cylinders in patients with corporal fibrosis. *Journal of Sexual Medicine* 3(4): 736–742.

[5] Jensen, JB., Larsen, EH., Kirkeby, HJ. & Jensen, KM. (2005). Clinical experience with the Mentor Alpha-1 inflatable penile prosthesis: Report on 65 patients. *Scandinavian Journal of Urology* 39(1): 69–72.

[6] Montorsi, F., Rigatti, P., Carmignani, G., Corbu, C., Campo, B., Ordesi, G., Breda, G., Silvestre, P., Giammusso, B., Morgia, G. & Graziottin, A. (2000). AMS three-piece inflatable implants for erectile dysfunction: a long-term multi-institutional study in 200 consecutive patients. *European Urology* 37(1): 50-55.

[7] Goldstein, I., Newman, L., Baum, N., Brooks, M., Chaikin, L., Goldberg, K., McBride, A. & Krane, RJ. (1997). Safety and efficacy outcome of mentor alpha-1 inflatable penile prosthesis implantation for impotence treatment. *Journal of Urology* 157(3): 833-839.

[8] Carson, CC., Mulcahy, JJ. & Govier, FE. (2000). Efficacy, safety and patient satisfaction outcomes of the AMS 700CX inflatable penile prosthesis: results of a long-term multicenter study. AMS 700CX Study Group. *Journal of Urology* 164(2): 376-380.

[9] Govier, FE., Gibbons, RP., Correa, RJ., Pritchett, TR. & Kramer-Levien, D. (1998). Mechanical reliability, surgical complications, and patient and partner satisfaction of the modern three-piece inflatable penile prosthesis. *Urology* 52(2): 282-286.

[10] Lee, SW., Park, BH., Lim, JH., Cui, WS., Kim, MK. & Park, JK. (2008). Prevention of urethral stricture in insertion of an inflatable penile prosthesis. *International Journal of Urology* 15(2): 162-165.

[11] Cui, WS., Kim, SD., Choi, KS., Zhao, C. & Park JK. (2009). An unusual success with simultaneous urethral repair and reimplantation of penile prosthesis in a patient with urethral stricture induced by rotated tubing. *Journal of Sexual Medicine* 6(6): 1783-1786.

[12] Cavalcanti, AG., Yucel, S., Deng, DY., McAninch, JW. & Baskin, LS. (2004). The distribution of neuronal and inducible nitric oxide synthase in urethral stricture formation. *Journal of Urology* 171(5): 1943-1947.

[13] Mundy, AR. & Andrich, DE. (2011). Urethral strictures. *British Journal of Urology International* 107(1): 6-26.

[14] Baskin, LS., Constantinescu, SC., Howard, PS., McAninch, JW., Ewalt, DH., Duckett, JW., Snyder, HM. & Macarak, EJ. (1993). Biochemical characterization and quantitation of the collagenous components of urethral stricture tissue. *Journal of Urology* 150(2): 642-647.

[15] Zhang, P., Shi, M., Wei, Q., Wang, K., Li, X., Li, H. & Bu, H. (2008). Increased expression of connective tissue growth factor in patients with urethral stricture. *Tohoku Journal of Experimental Medicine* 215(3): 199–206.

[16] Fenton, AS., Morey, AF., Aviles, R. & Garcia, CR. (2005). Anterior urethral strictures: etiology and characteristics. *Urology* 65(6): 1055-1058.

10

Genital Skin Flap Urethroplasty

Abimbola O. Olajide
Ladoke Akintola University of Technology
Nigeria

1. Introduction

Urethral stricture disease is one of the commonest diseases treated by Urologists. No two forms of the disease can be assumed to be the same because of the varied aetiologies and modalities of management. Choice of treatment modality depends on location of the stricture, available facilities and the experience of the managing surgeon.

Urethral dilatation and internal urethrotomy as modalities of treatment have limited usage in current day practice because when there is associated spongiofibrosis, they are not curative. Urethral reconstruction has therefore become the mainstay treatment of urethral stricture disease when the aim is to cure the patient of such a crippling ailment. (Rosen et al., 1994) Anastomotic urethroplasty is considered the best form of reconstruction when possible because no tissue can replace the urethra better then the urethra itself. (Santucci et al., 2002) However, anastomotic urethroplasty has limited application in urethral reconstruction because it can cause abnormal penile curvature (chordee) due to shortening of the urethra relative to the spongy tissues during penile erection. This may result in painful erection and disturbance of sexual function with resultant psychological disturbances. Anastomotic urethroplasty is therefore better avoided in reconstruction of some urethral stricture like those located in the penile urethra or long segment stricture (>2cm) located in the bulbar urethra. In such cases, substitution urethroplasty is considered most appropriate. (Kellner et al., 2004) Since its introduction, substitution urethroplasty has remained one of the standard methods for urethral reconstruction especially in difficult urethral stricture or where other modalities of treatment have failed. (Olajide et al., 2010)

Several tissues have been used to replace diseased urethra and the best tissue to use is an area of controversy. Buccal mucosa, bladder mucosa, intestinal mucosa, scrotal skin, perineal skin and penile skin are some of the tissues that have been used. Some are used as graft while others are used as flaps. However, one incontrovertible finding is the fact that flaps have an obvious advantage over grafts because it does not depend on the blood supply of the recipient tissue which may be non dependable in some situation because of associated severe spongiofibrosis and precarious blood supply. (MacDonald & Santucci, 2005)

2. Classification of genital skin

Although there is no conventional classification of the genital skin in the literature, with regards to urethral reconstruction, genital skin can be classified into the hirsute (hair bearing) and the non-hirsute (non-hair bearing). This is necessary because the presence or absence of hair is taken into consideration in the choice of genital skin to use as the consequences of hair within the urethra could be crippling. All the skin around the external genitalia have been tried in urethral reconstruction at different stages in the evolution of substitution urethroplasty, these include the perineal, scrotal, penile and preputial skin.

2.1 Hirsute skin

Scrotal and perineal skin were used for urethral reconstruction in the past but the outcome was not favourable. (Mundy, 1993, 1995) Despite the close proximity to the urethra, the pedicle is often short and the flap doesn't go farther than the bulbar urethra. The greatest problem with such flaps is the presence of hair with complications such as obstruction to flow of urine, recurrent urinary tract infection and urethral calculi formation. (Crew et al., 1996) This equally applies to the proximal penile skin which is hair bearing and therefore avoided when constructing penile skin flap. This explains the limitation of flap length with longitudinal distal penile skin flap: the longer the flap length, the more the risk of harvesting hair bearing proximal penile skin. Attempt was made at pre-operative depilation using laser or electrocautery but the outcome remains disappointing (Finkelstein & Blatstein, 1991). Since understanding the fact that urethral hair growth is inevitable sequelae of using hair bearing skin for urethral reconstruction, use of scrotal and perineal skin has been abandoned.

2.2 Non-hirsute skin

Non-hirsute genital skin includes the preputial and distal penile skin. These have been used with remarkable successes recorded by all. Currently, non-hirsute genital skin has become a 'formidable weapon' in the hand of seasoned urologists to cure the menace of urethral stricture worldwide. The skin is hairless, adapted to wetness and enough to be closed back without tension after removal of part of it.

3. Advantages of genital skin flap

Advantages of genital skin flap for urethral reconstruction are numerous and it has been found very versatile in all forms of anterior urethral reconstruction. The skin and its superficial fascia have generous blood supply from the external pudendal artery which is a branch of the femoral artery. Therefore, when raised as a flap, the penile skin is able to support itself without dependence on the blood supply of the corpus spongiosum which is the recipient tissue. This explains why this tissue survives when the prevailing conditions in the recipient site is unfavourable, e.g. in the presence of fibrosis and/or wound infection, or when grafts have failed. Furthermore, the underlying superficial fascia containing the blood vessels can be easily raised from the underlying deep fascia as the pedicle of the flap. When properly done, this pedicle can be long enough to reach any part of the urethra, from the prostatic portion to the meatus. Proximity of the genital skin to the urethra makes it possible to carry out the reconstruction as a single procedure by flipping it over to the adjacent urethra to replace the strictured segment. (Elliot & McAninch, 2008)
The preputial / penile skin is relatively thin, pliable and able to withstand prolonged contact with urine than most other tissues. Enough skin can also be raised as flap from this source to substitute the whole anterior urethra. More so, being hairless, the fear of hair ball formation, recurrent infection or urethral calculi from hair growth within the lumen is

excluded (Hinman Jr., 1991). Genital skin flap can be used as an onlay or tubularised to substitute the entire circumference of a urethral segment and the donor site heals perfectly with barely noticeable scar. This is because the incisions are made along pre-existing or natural skin lines like the circumcision line or the median raphe on the ventral surface of the penis. There is therefore neither cosmetic nor psychological problem arising from the post operative scar. (Elliot & McAninch, 2008)
Lastly, the procedure can be done under regional techniques of anaesthesia like spinal or epidural block. This is possible because both the donor and the recipient sites are in the same region of the body and supplied by similar nerve roots. Thus, general anaesthesia and its attendant complications can be avoided.

4. Limitations of genital skin flap

Lichen Sclerosis of the penile skin (Balanitis Xerotica Obliterans) is a chronic progressive disease of the genital skin which may be responsible for urethral stricture disease itself. The aetiology is unknown and there is no satisfactory treatment till date. It causes white patches on the skin which later becomes atrophic and hardened. When this affects the genital skin or if it is the cause of the urethral stricture, it makes the skin unusable for urethral reconstruction. (Barbagli et al., 2004) Where a patient has had previous hypospadias repair complicated by urethral stricture, the penile skin is of poor quality because of the cicatrisation from previous surgery. (Imamoglu et al., 2003) Such a skin is not ideal for substitution of the urethra. Rarely, recurrent balanitis/balanoposthitis with scarring or perforation of the preputial skin may make the skin unusable for reconstruction. Preputial skin may be unavailable if the patient has had circumcision prior to presentation. In such situation, distal penile skin can still be used if it is adjudged normal and unlikely to be involved in the primary pathology. (Quartey, 1987)

5. Applied anatomy of penis

Good understanding of the anatomy of penis and its covering is an important prerequisite to successful construction of preputial or distal penile island skin flap for urethral substitution. This is because construction of these flaps is based on the natural relatively bloodless planes of the superficial fascia of the penis. Furthermore, penile skin flaps used in urethral reconstruction are 'axial' (based on definite vessel) and 'island' (completely detached from the skin from which it is raised); they are only attached by the pedicle which contains the vascular supply to the island of skin. (Tung & Nichols, 2008) Thus, understanding of the distribution and location of the vessels are important for successful creation of such flap for reconstruction of the urethra.

5.1 Structure of penis

The penis is composed of three cylindrical erectile tissues: 2 paired corpora carvernosa dorsally and a corpus spongiosum located ventrally in the groove between the corpora carvernosa. These erectile tissues are made up of blood spaces lined by endothelium and each is enclosed by a tough, fibrous-elastic capsule called tunica albuginea. (Figure I) Corpora carvernosa bodies are fused together in the midline, separated only by an incomplete septum, while corpus spongiosum contains the urethra within it. At the distal end of the penis, corpus spongiosum expands to form the glans which is folded proximally to cover the distal ends of the corpora cavernosa. Proximally, the corpora carvernosa bodies separate as they approach the perineum to become the crura which are covered by the ischiocarvernosus muscles and attached to the medial margins of the ischio-pubic bone. The corpus spongiosum at this region becomes expanded to form the bulb which is surrounded by the bulbospongiosus muscle and together are attached to the inferior surface of the urogenital diaphragm. The urethra within the bulb makes an upward bend through the urogenital diaphragm to become the membranous urethra. Superficial to the tunica albuginea of the erectile bodies is the deep fascia of the penis called "Buck's Fascia". It forms a common covering for the corpus spongiosum and the two corpora carvernosa. It is closely adherent to the tunica albuginea which makes it difficult to separate. Beneath this fascia, in the groove between the two corpora cavernosa lie deep dorsal vein, dorsal arteries and the dorsal nerve which supplies the deep structures of the penis. Outside this fascia lie the loose areolar subcutaneous tissue (dartos) and the skin.

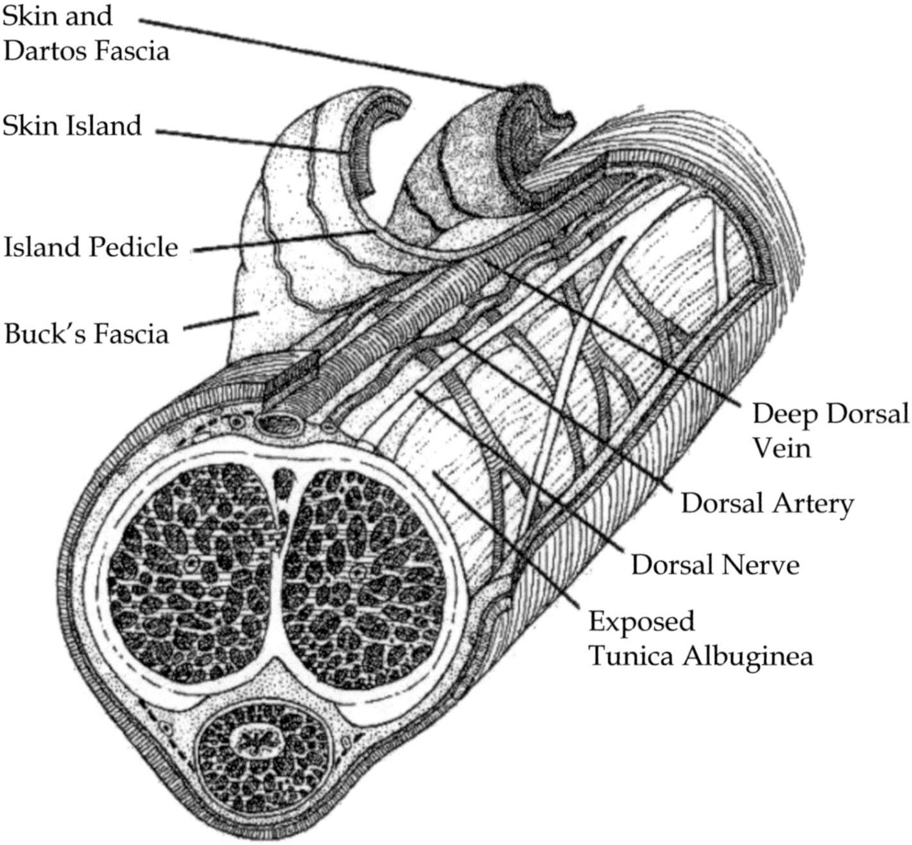

Fig. 1. Structure of penis and its coverings. (From Buckley & Mc Aninch, 2007)

5.2 Coverings of penis (skin and subcutaneous tissue)

The dartos fascia is devoid of fat, slides freely over the underlying Buck's fascia and continuous with membranous layer of the superficial fascia (Scarpa's fascia) of the anterior abdominal wall. It can be separated into two layers with the superficial layer closely apposed to the skin of the penis while the deeper layer contains the superficial vessels, nerves and lymphatics of the penis. (Figure 1) They are termed dartos fascia and tunica dartos respectively. (Buckley & MacAninch 2007) The skin is the outermost covering of penis. It is thin, devoid of fat and loose with non prominent smooth muscle fibre (dartos muscle) in the dermis which allows the skin to accommodate changes in the size of the penis when flaccid or turgid. Below the dermis is a subdermal vascular plexus which is supplied by the superficial branches of external pudendal vessels given off at the root of the penis. During dissection to create the flap, care must be taken to preserve the subdermal plexus so that necrosis of penile skin does not occur. The skin and dartos fascia of the penis are prolonged as a double layer from the coronal sulcus, covering the glans to a variable extent. This is the prepuce of the penis. It is essentially a folding of the penile skin on itself, which is stretched to a single layer during penile erection and by retraction over the penile shaft. The outer surface of the prepuce is normal skin but the inner surface is mucosal membrane; although it resembles skin in appearance, there is a muco-cutaneous boundary just inside the tip of the prepuce. The entire skin system moves freely due a low friction gliding plane immediately beneath the surface of the skin, thus the skin of the penis does not adhere to the underlying tissue the way skin adheres in other parts of the body. This skin can move as a unit back and forth longitudinally or around the shaft circumferentially making it the most mobile skin in male. These qualities make the penile skin redundant and afford easy closure after a portion of it is removed as flap.

5.3 Vascular supply

The deep structures are supplied by internal pudendal artery which runs beneath the buck's fascia while the skin and superficial fascia are supplied by the superficial and deep external pudendal arteries which are branches of the femoral arteries. After branching from femoral artery, these vessels run medially towards the penis in the membranous layer of the superficial fascia. (Figure 2)

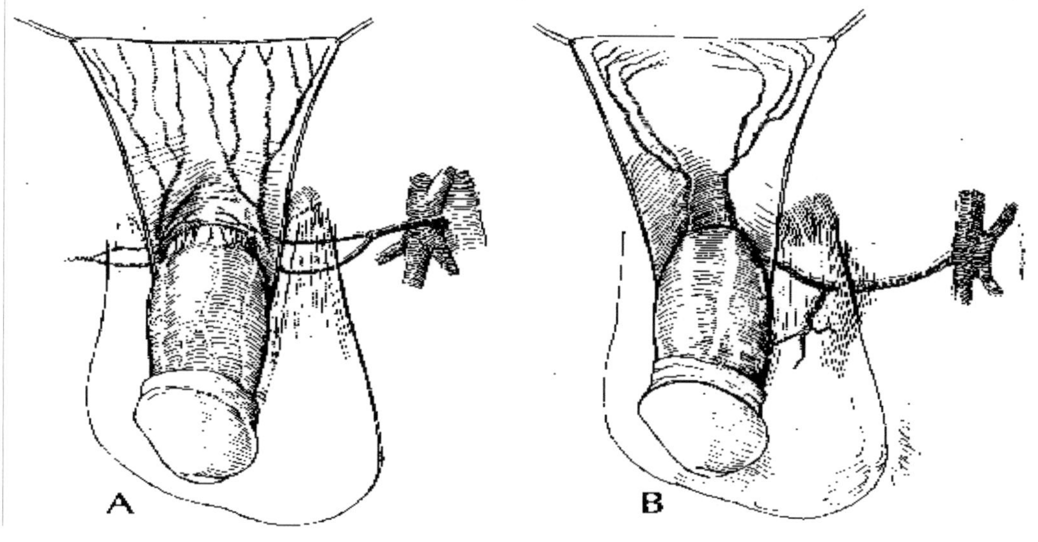

Fig. 2. Arterial supply and venous drainage of penile coverings (From Hinman Jr, 1991)

At the base of the penis, they divide into dorsolateral and ventrolateral axial penile branches which run distally in the tunica dartos of the subcutaneous tissue, dividing into smaller branches which ramify to cover the entire skin and the superficial facia of the penis. At the base of the penis, they give superficial branches which supply the subdermal plexus of vessels. The prepuce being a double layer of skin has a single terminal arterial system, axially oriented in the subcutaneous tissue such that after retraction, the vessels are seen to end at the coronal sulcus and not at the preputial ring. The venous drainage follows the arterial pattern with venae comitantes accompanying the arteries. At the root of the penis, a small venous trunk emerges from the subdermal plexus to join the venae comitantes which ultimately drains into the femoral vein.

Principle of developing preputial/distal penile skin flap requires two planes of dissection: superficially between the dartos fascia and tunica dartos (sub-epithelial plane) and deeper between the tunica dartos and buck's fascia (sub-dartos plane). These are relatively avascular planes which make it easy to separate the skin with the adherent dartos fascia from the tunica dartos and also to separate the tunica dartos from the underlying buck's fascia. The tunica dartos with its rich vascular supply forms the pedicle which carries the blood supply to the island of penile or preputial skin to be used for reconstruction. (Brandes, 2008)

6. Applications of penile/preputial skin flap in urethroplasty

Penile skin island flaps are versatile, and applicable in all forms of anterior urethral reconstruction irrespective of the location, length and number of stricture. In the hand of an experienced urologist, the long term success rate is encouraging. Though it is technically challenging, knowledge of the anatomy of penis and adherence to basic principles of tissue transfer are fundamental to the successes recorded with these methods. (Brandes, 2008) Penile skin flaps are used in congenital conditions like hypospadias and congenital strictures. They are also used in acquired conditions like urethral stricture diseases especially when options are limited due to the complex nature of the diseases or unfavourable conditions of the recipient site like infection or precarious blood supply due to extensive fibrosis.

The goal of urethral reconstruction for stricture can be summarise by the following three points:

- Removal of obstruction i.e. resolution of the pre-operative symptoms and prevention of possible sequelae.
- Cosmetically acceptable appearance of the penis after the procedure.
- Normal sexual intercourse i.e. absence of chordee and no pain on erection or sexual intercourse.

These are all taken care of by the use of the genital skin flaps because adequate skin can be harvested as flap to maintain adequate urethral length and prevent chordee while skin incisions are created along pre-existing skin lines (median raphe and/or circumcision line) to give cosmetically acceptable scar.

Various techniques abound in the literature but all the techniques using penile skin flaps are based on same principle with differences being only in the orientation of the flap (transversely or longitudinally), or whether raised ventrally or dorsally. (Jordan & Rourke, 2006) These basic principles will be described using 3 techniques: Transverse preputial island flap, transverse distal penile island flap, and longitudinal distal penile island flap.

6.1 Transverse distal penile island flap

6.1.1 Indication

More suitable for long segment stricture (>2cm) of the bulbar urethra, when the prepuce in unavailable or not usable. Although more technically difficult than the longitudinal distal penile island flap, it can also be used for penile urethral stricture. It has also been applied in the repair of posterior urethral stricture. (Quartey, 1987)

6.1.2 Recommended instruments

Ring retractor or Turner-Warwick perineal retractor, van Burren (antegrade) sound, fine serrated scissors, bipolar electrocautery, non crushing forceps.

6.1.3 Pre-operative preparation

Retrograde urethrogram with or without micturating urethrogram is done to know the site and length of the stricture and to guide the surgeon intra-operatively. Urethral ultrasonography may be done to know the extent and depth of involvement of the spongy tissue. A fleet enema can be given on the evening before surgery to avoid bowel motion in the immediate post operative period which could lead to wound infection. The skin of the perineum is shaved preferably on the morning of surgery and the genitalia and perineum washed with soap and copious amount of water to reduce bacterial load. Prophylactic intravenous quinolone and metronidazole is given just before anaesthesia is administered.

6.1.4 Anaesthesia and position

Spinal or epidural block can be used when not contraindicated. This is one of the advantages of using the genital flap over extra-genital graft since the spinal block also anaesthetizes the donor area. In few selected patients, we have done this procedure under saddle block with good intra and post operative outcome.
Where spinal or epidural block is contraindicated or when patient refuses them, a general anaesthesia can also be used. However, in the paediatric age group, general anaesthesia is always used.

6.1.5 Position

Lithotomy position is used in distal bulbar stricture. When the lesion is in the proximal bulbar region, an exaggerated lithotomy is preferred to aid exposure.

6.1.6 Procedure

Following anaesthesia and positioning, the skin is prepped and drapped to expose the perineum, external genitalia and suprapubic region (Figure 3). If the patient does not have suprapubic cystostomy prior surgery, one is created before perineal incision. This allows for passage of antegrade sound to delineate the proximal end of the stricture. A size 18FG Foley's catheter is also passed retrogradely through the urethra to delineate the distal end of the stricture. An inverted 'Y' incision is made on the perineum with the vertical part on the median raphe extending from the perineo-scrotal junction to about 2.5cm from the anus. The wings of the 'Y' are carried on either sides of the anus to a point medial to the ischial tuberosity. The incision is deepened in the midline through the colle's fascia to expose bulbospongiosus muscle (Figure 4), which is then incised in the midline to expose the bulbar urethra and the bulb. The bulb is mobilised by separating the muscles laterally and the corpora cavernosa dorsally. Care should be taken at the proximal end of the bulb where the arteries to the bulb enter laterally. Inadvertent division of these vessels at this stage could result in severe haemorrhage due to the limited operating space, the shortness of the vessels and retraction when divided. Mobilization of the urethra at the region of the stricture may be very difficult because of the surrounding spongiofibrosis, it is thus easier and better to start mobilization from the normal urethral (distally) where the dissection planes are preserved. Care should be taken not to take the distal dissection beyond the suspensory ligament to prevent chordee post operatively. The dissection is continued proximally, mobilising the strictured segment of the urethra completely until normal urethral proximally. Urethrotomy incision is then made through the dorsal or ventral surface into the lumen of the urethra (Figure 5), extending 0.5-1cm into the normal urethra proximally and distally to prevent stricture recurrence. The length and width of the flap to be constructed is then measure before proceeding to its construction. The perineal wound is packed with gauze to reduce haemorrhage from the corpus spongiosum while constructing the skin flap.

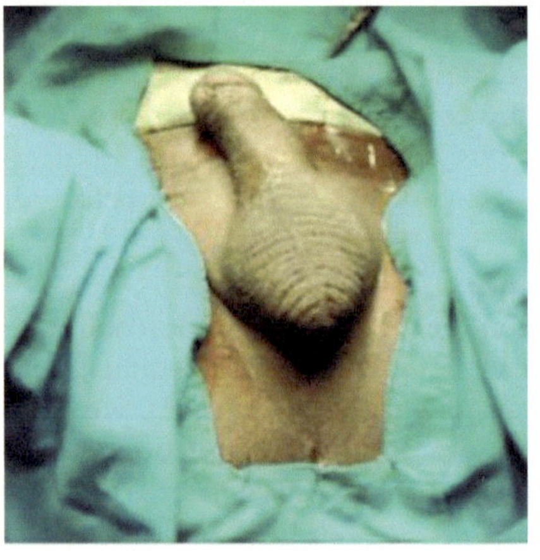

Fig. 3. Skin draped to expose the operation site

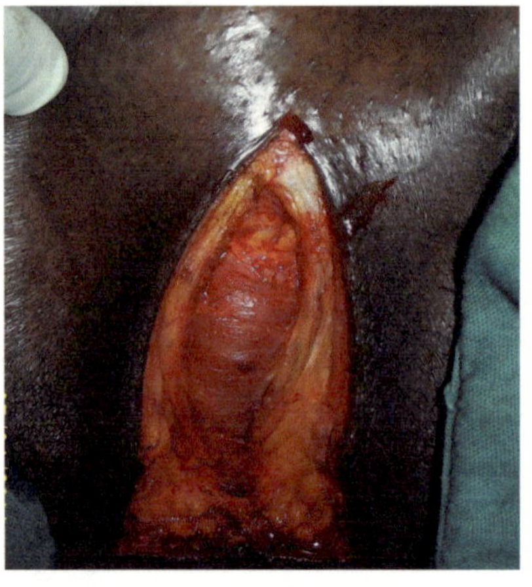

Fig. 4. Inverted "Y" perineal incision deepened through subcutaneous layer to expose the bulbospongiosus muscle

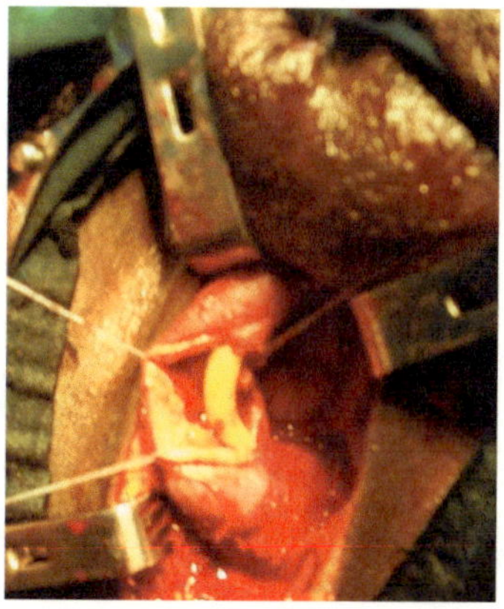

Fig. 5. Incision of the dorsal aspect of the urethra (urethrotomy) exposing the strictured region of the urethra

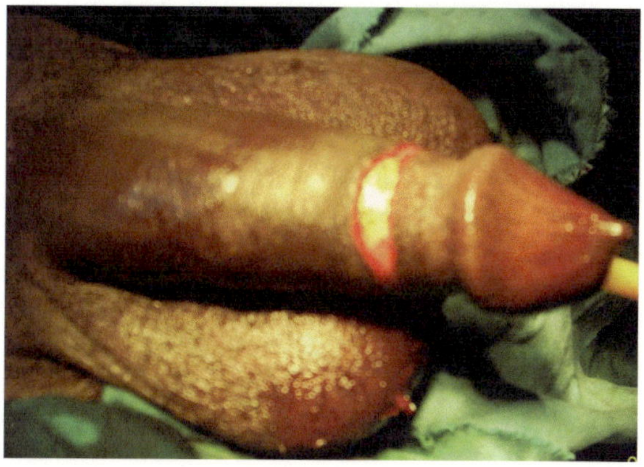

Fig. 6. Circumferential skin incision along the circumcision line, deepened to the avascular plane between the tunica dartos and Buck's fascia

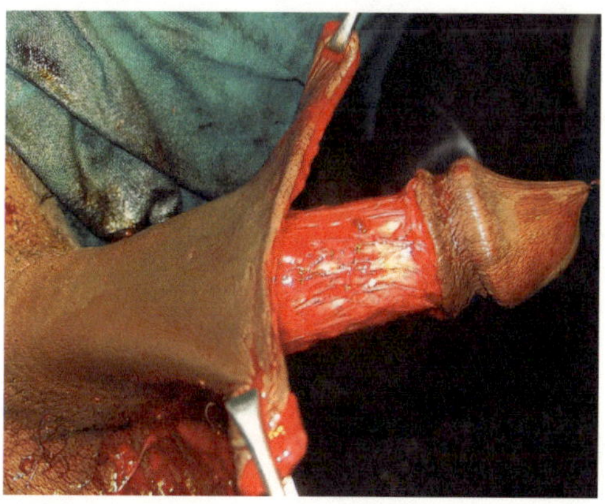

Fig. 7. De-gloved penis with its covering opened like a sheet by longitudinal extension of incision along median raphe

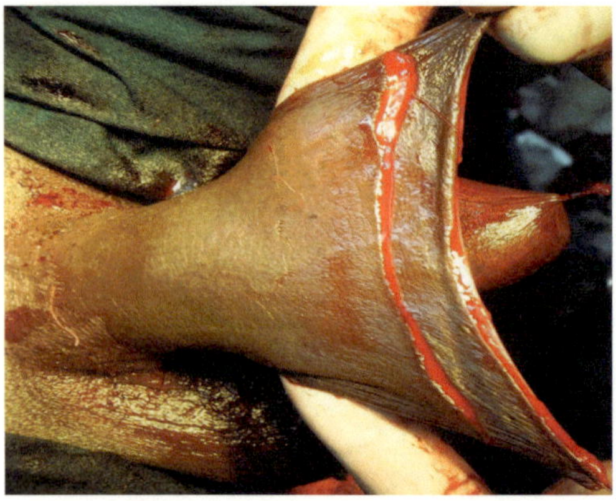

Fig. 8. Second skin incision deepened to the avascular plane between the dartos fascia and the tunica dartos, mapping the island of skin for reconstruction

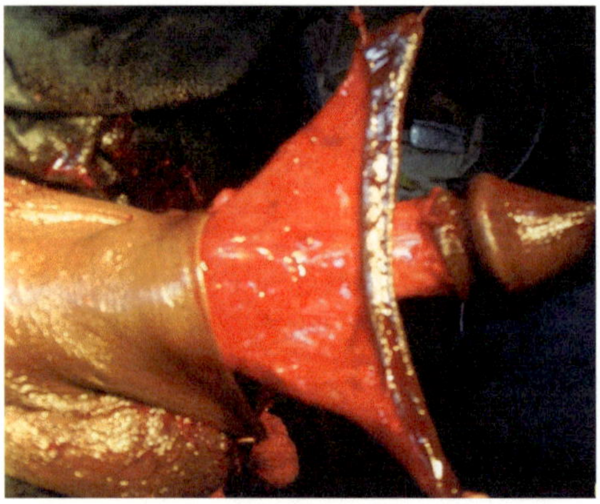

Fig. 9. Island of skin to be used for reconstruction with its pedicle

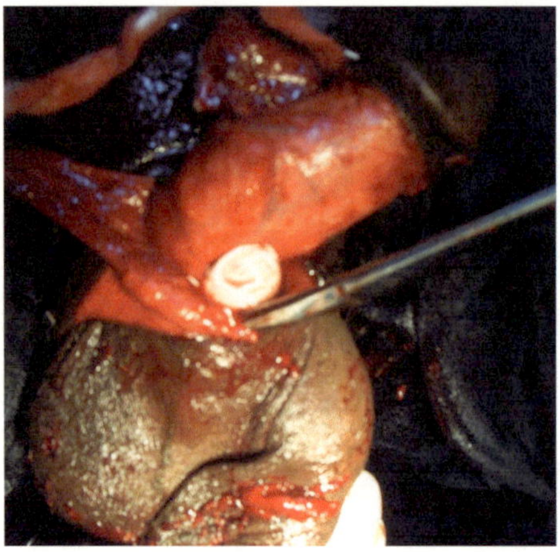

Fig. 10. Creation of retro-scrotal tunnel through which the island and its pedicle is delivered into the perineum

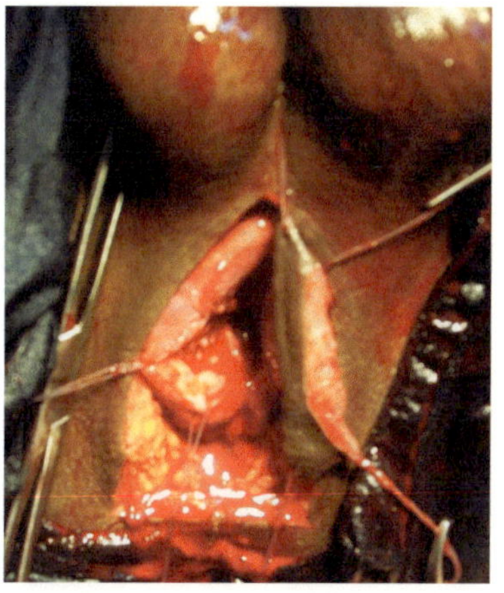

Fig. 11. Skin Island already delivered into the perineum

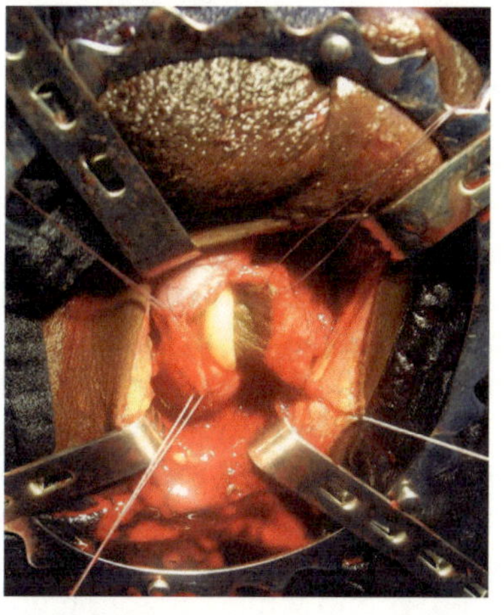

Fig. 12. Anastomosis of the skin island to the urethra with Foley's catheter in the lumen

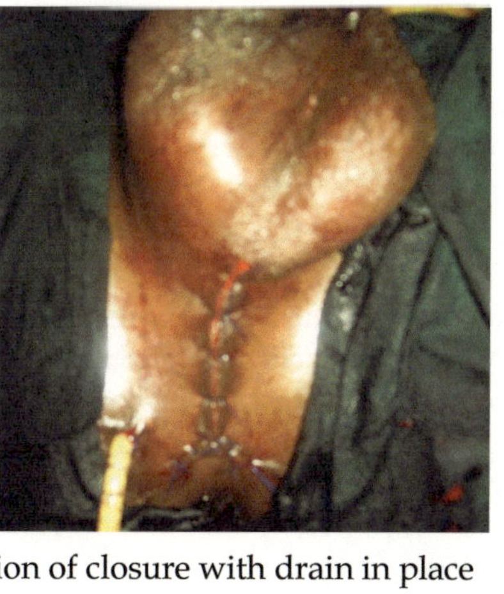

Fig. 13. Perineum on completion of closure with drain in place

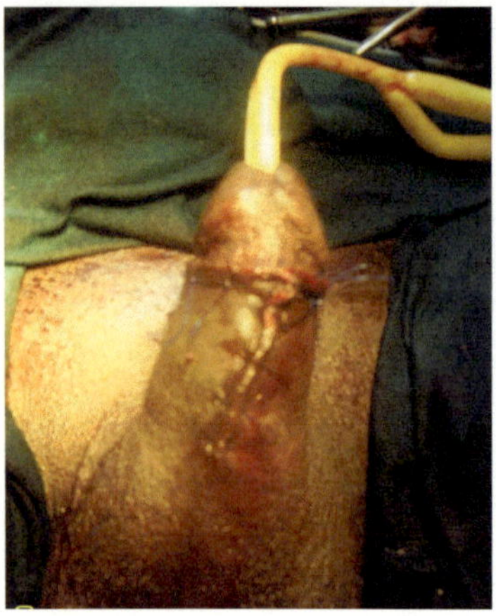

Fig. 14. Penis after closure of the skin

A 2/0 silk suture is used as stay on the glans penis to keep the penis extended while dissection is going on. A circumferential incision is made just proximal to the coronal sulcus on the penile skin and deepened to the buck's fascia (Figure 6). On the midline ventrally (on median raphe), the incision is extended proximally to the penoscrotal junction. A plane is created between the tunica dartos and the buck's fascia through which the penis is degloved by combination of both blunt and sharp dissection to the root of the penis (Figure 7). Starting from the frenular end, another incision that is skin-deep is made proximal to the initial incision to map out the island of skin to be used for the reconstruction. The distance between the two incisions should equal the width of the urethral gap to be bridged (Figure 8). The second incision is deepened just to the plane between the dartos fascia and the tunica dartos, where the penile skin and the firmly adherent dartos facia is carefully dissected off the tunica dartos which contains the vascular supply to the island skin flap. Care must be taken to preserve the subdermal plexus and avoid necrosis of the penile skin (Figure 9). A tunnel is created deep to the scrotum by insinuating the index finger from the perineal wound below, towards the penile wound while dissecting with scissors from above to meet the insinuating finger (Figure 10). Through this retroscrotal tunnel, the island flap is delivered into the perineum (Figure 11). Care is taking to avoid twisting of the pedicle at this stage so that the vascular supply of the flap is not compromised. Excess skin can be trimmed off to prevent redundant skin which could lead to diverticulum as the flap is sutured as onlay to the native urethra to bridge the gap using a 5-0 polyglycolic or polyglactin interrupted suture (Figure 12). Care should also taken to ensure that the knots of the suture are outside the lumen. After completion of one side of the anastomosis, a size 16FG or 18FG Foley's catheter is passed through the urethra into the bladder to serve as stent for the repair. A wound drain is sometimes placed underneath the bulbospongiosus muscle if there is extensive dissection around the scrotum or if there is significant oozing of blood from the dissected spongiofibrosis. The drain is brought out through a stab wound on the skin of the perineum, aimed at preventing hematoma collection when this is anticipated (Figure 13). The incision is closed in layers and firm sterile pressure dressing is applied sparing the anus. Suprapubic catheter is placed in the cystostomy site for diversion of urine and penile skin closure is done with interrupted 3-0 nylon suture (Figure 14). An occlusive dressing is also applied to the penis.

Where there is a long segment stricture with completely occluded lumen precluding onlay repair, the urethral segment can be excised and the flap tubularised around a catheter which is then sutured to the proximal and distal urethral to bridge the gap. However, the success rate for tubularisation of the flap is lower when compared with onlay repair. (Carney & McAninch, 2002) Thus, onlay repair is favoured by most urologists when intraoperative findings allow it.

6.1.7 Post operative management

Intravenous antibiotics and analgesics are continued for 24-48 hours and changed to oral thereafter. Perineal wound drain, if placed, is removed on the second or third post operative day and the penile occlusive dressing is changed on the fourth or fifth day after inspection of both wounds.

Perineal and penile stitches are removed between the eighth and tenth day. Pericatheter urethrogram is done 14-21 days after surgery, following which the catheter is removed if there is no extravasation of contrast. Uroflowmetry is done at varied interval to assess the urine flow rate.

6.1.8 Complications

Common early post operative complications are wound infection, urosepsis, urethrocutaneous fistula, scrotal haematoma, penile skin necrosis, epididymo-orchitis and flap necrosis. Late complications include urethral diverticulum and restenosis of the urethra.

6.2 Transverse preputial island flap

The inner surface (mucosa) of the preputial skin is preferred for reasons explained earlier. Where the prepuce is intact, this technique should be chosen, but where the patient is circumcised, distal penile skin is considered.

6.2.1 Indication

Use of preputial island flap was initially described and has been widely used in the repair of all forms of hypospadias with or without chordee. Its use is however not limited to hypospadias as it has been applied to reconstruction of the urethra for various forms of stricture disease. In uncircumcised adult, it has been widely used in reconstruction of urethra stricture located any part of the urethra, even membranous urethra. Application of this method for hypospadias is not described in this chapter.

6.2.2 Recommended instruments

Ring retractor or Turner-Warwick perineal retractor, van-Burren (antegrade) sound, fine serrated scissors, bipolar electrocautery, non crushing forceps.

6.2.3 Pre-operative preparation

Delineation of stricture length and location by retrograde urethrogram with or without micturating urethrogram is essential. Urethral ultrasound may also be used to characterise the strictured segment and the surrounding tissue. On the morning of surgery, perineum and external genitalia is shaved and washed thoroughly with soap and copious amount of water, prepuce is retracted and the inner skin is similarly washed to reduce bacterial load. A fleet enema is given on the evening before surgery to avoid bowel motion in the immediate post operative period. Prophylactic intravenous quinolone and metronidazole is given just before anaesthesia.

6.2.4 Anaesthesia

Just like for transverse distal penile island flap, spinal or epidural block can be used. Where these regional block methods cannot be used because it is contraindicated or because the patient prefers not to be conscious during the surgery, general anaesthesia can also be used. In contrary, when this procedure is done in paediatric age group for hypospadias or any other urethral pathology, general anaesthesia is always used.

6.2.5 Position

Lithotomy or exaggerated lithotomy as explained under the transverse distal penile island flap repair.

6.2.6 Proceedure

The steps in exposure of the diseased bulbar urethra are as described for transverse distal penile island flap urethroplasty. The main technical difference in the two procedure is the need to retract the prepuce over the penile shaft before raising the flap form the inner preputial skin.
A 2/0 silk penile suture is placed at the dorsum of the glans to allow for traction on the penis while dissection is ongoing. The prepuce is retracted back and pulled on the penile shaft so that the two layers of skin becomes single and continuous around the penile shaft. A circumferential incision is made 0.5-1.0 cm proximal to the corona, this is deepened to subdartos plane just as explained for the distal penile island flap. The penis is degloved at this avascular plane up to the root of the penis; the incision is then extended down vertically on the midline (median raphe) on the ventral surface of the penis such that the penile/preputial skin can be opened out as a flat sheet of skin rather than a circumferential one. A transverse island flap from the inner layer of the prepuce is outlined with another proximal skin incision, deepened to the plane between the fascia dartos and tunica dartos. The dimensions of this island of skin is also measured based on the size needed to cover the defect in the urethral without redundancy. The skin and the fascia Dartos are carefully dissected off the underlying tunica dartos which is the pedicle containing the vascular supply to the flap. The flap with its axial vascular pedicle is dissected proximally up to the root of penis to allow ventral transposition of the island flap with no tension. A retroscrotal tunnel is created and the island flap is delivered into the perineal wound for anastomosis to bridge the urethral gap.

6.2.7 Post operative management

This is essentially as described for the transverse distal penile island flap method.

6.2.8 Complications

Complications of this technique are similar to those described for transverse distal penile island flap. However; flap necrosis is theoretically more likely than distal penile island flap because of longer length of pedicle and smaller size of vessels supplying the preputial skin.

6.3 Longitudinal distal penile island flap

6.3.1 Indications

Whenever stricture involves the penile urethra, anastomotic urethroplasty is not favoured because it can cause unacceptable penile deformity on erection, thereby putting sexual function at risk. Substitution urethroplasty is therefore the mainstay of reconstruction in penile urethral stricture. Longitudinal distal penile island flap is technically easier and faster than the transverse distal penile island flap in the repair of penile urethral stricture.

6.3.2 Recommended instruments

Fine serrated scissors, non-crushing forceps, bipolar electrocautery.

6.3.3 Pre-operative preparation

The strictured segment is characterised using ultrasonography and urethrography. The non hirsute region of the penile skin can be marked before shaving or else the penile skin is not shaved to allow the surgeon to mark a flap without incorporating hair. Penile skin can be washed with soap on the morning of surgery to reduce the load of microorganism. Peri-operative quinolone and metronidazole are given just before anaesthesia.

6.3.4 Anaesthesia

Spinal or epidural block is preferred though general anaesthesia can also be used.

6.3.5 Position

Supine position is preferred for penile urethral reconstruction.

6.3.6 Procedure

Following spinal or epidural block and positioning, the skin is prepped and draped to expose the penis and suprapubic region. A 2-0 silk suture is applied to the glans for traction and a size 18 FG Foley's catheter passed through the meatus to mark the distal end of the stricture. A curvilinear skin incision is made on one side of the midline on the ventral surface of the penis, deepened through the dartos layer and buck's fascia onto the tunica albuginea of the corpus cavernosum. The edge of the skin is elevated and dissected across the midline to the other corpus cavernosum to expose the strictured segment of the urethra. Longitudinal urethrotomy incision is then made on the urethra to expose the lumen of the strictured segment. This is done on the lateral surface of the urethra opposite to side of the skin incision and extending about 1 cm into the normal urethra proximally and distally. The size 18 FG Foley's catheter is advanced proximally in the urethra to assess the remaining part of the urethra for stricture (Figure 15). The length and width of the flap needed to complete the circumference of the urethra is measured once the diseased segment is laid open. The partially raised flap is marked based on the dimension of the strictured segment and another incision made through the skin, deepened to the plane between the Darto's fascia and tunica Dartos, outlining the island flap to be constructed for the repair. Blunt and sharp dissections are carried out on this plane to isolate the marked skin on the vascular pedicle made of tunica Dartos (Figure 16). Care must be taken at this level to ensure dissection is done at the proper plane to preserve the subdermal plexus and prevent necrosis of the penile skin being raised form the tunica dartos. The skin flap is rotated into the urethral defect and a watertight anastomosis is done with interrupted 5-0 polyglycolic or polyglactin suture, ensuring that knots are extra-luminal. Size i6 or 18 FG Foley's catheter is left in place to serve as a stent (Figure 17). This small size catheter is actually preferred to allow drainage of secretions or blood around the catheter and to prevent pressure necrosis of urethral mucosa due to large catheter which could result in another stricture at a later date.

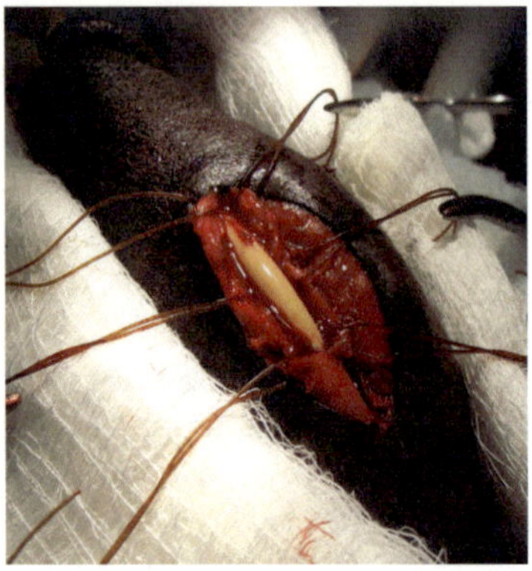

Fig. 15. Urethrotomy incision into the strictured segment of the urethra

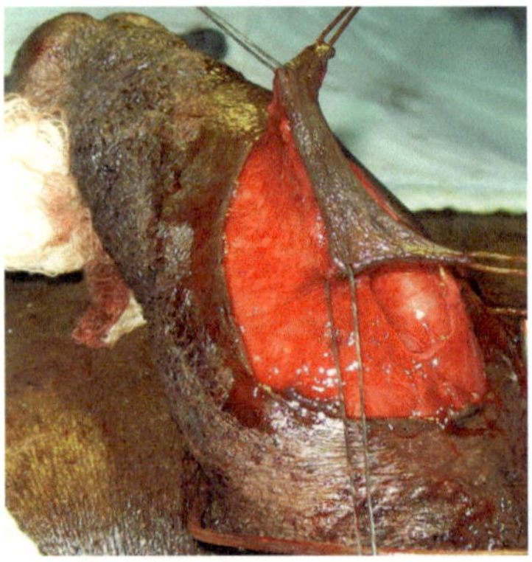

Fig. 16. Longitudinal island flap constructed on its pedicle

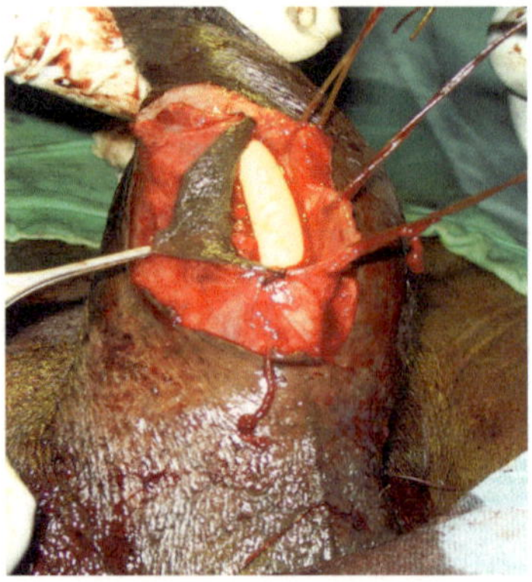

Fig. 17. Anastomosis of the island flap to the native urethra

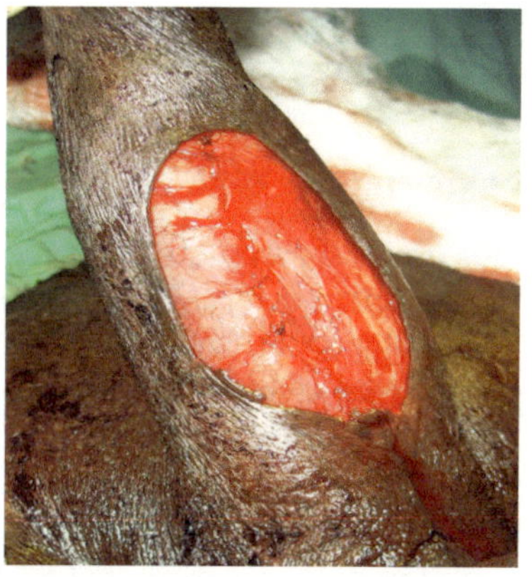

Fig. 18. Completed of anastomosis

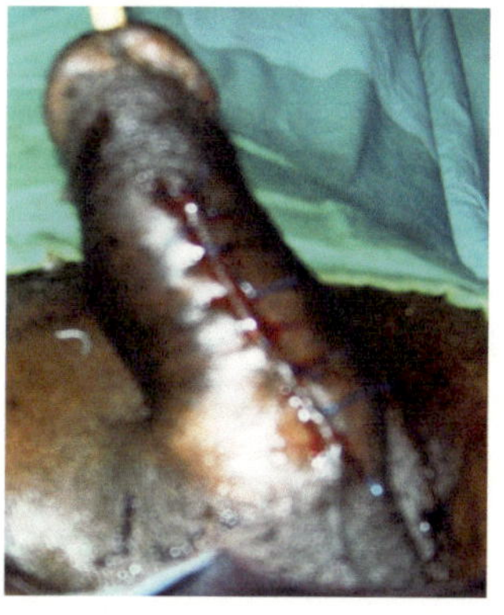

Fig. 19. Final appearance of penis on completion of repair

A layer of subcutaneous (dartos) fascia can be closed over the anastomosis before penile skin closure with interrupted 3-0 nylon suture. Patients with pre-operative suprapubic cystostomy are maintained on diversion by inserting Foley's catheter into the suprapubic opening while those without suprapubic cystostomy are left un-diverted. An occlusive dressing is applied with the penis retracted dorsally and anchored to the anterior abdominal wall to reduce oedema.

6.3.7 Post operative management

Intravenous antibiotics and analgesics are continued for 24-48 hours and changed to oral drugs thereafter. Wound is inspected on the third or fourth post operative day and dressing is changed. Stitches are removed after 7-10 days and peri-catheter urethrogram is done 14-21 days after surgery, following which the catheter is removed if there is no extravasation. Uroflowmetry can be after 3 months to evaluate the urine flow.

6.3.8 Complications

Urethrocutaneous fistula can result but usually resolves within few days. Wound infection and penile skin necrosis are not common if the surgeon adheres to basic rules of raising flaps. Recurrence is rarely seen if the strictured segment was properly laid open during surgery. Hair in the urethra could occur if a long flap extending to the hirsuite proximal penile skin is used to construct the flap for a long segment stricture.

7. Experience with genital skin flap

We have used genital skin flap for urethral reconstruction in our unit and have found it very useful in complex cases of urethral stricture. Between 2002 and 2008, we treated about 55 cases with success rate of 81.2% (Olajide et al, 2010). Commonest early post operative complication was wound infection which was not surprising because a large proportion of the patient had significant bacteriuria pre-operatively. Commonest delayed complication was urethral diverticulum which made us to trim our flap more thereafter and to use dorsal urethrotomy and dorsal onlay anastomosis which is associated with lesser occurrence of diverticulum. Recurrence was found in only one patient (1.8%) 2 years post operation.

Preputial island flap in our unit is practiced mainly for hypospadias because circumcision is practiced routinely in Nigeria for religious and cultural reasons. Virtually all our patients are circumcised; this fact negates the use of prepuce for urethral reconstruction in adult in out unit. We reported use of this flap for hypospadias 2009, (Sowande et al, 2009) but this experience cannot be extrapolated to the adult because they are treating different clinical conditions.

Longitudinal penile island flap is routinely used in our unit to treat all strictures located in the penile urethra. Though yet unpublished, we treated 23 cases over a 4 year period and found penile skin necrosis in 2 patients which healed on wound dressing. All the patients had satisfactory outcome.

8. Future trend

Introduction of vascularised flap techniques and use of grafts has broadened the field of urethral reconstruction. Several modifications of the original techniques have evolved and more are still on the way. With improvement in immune modulation and techniques of tissue transfer, substitution with both allogeneic, xenogeneic and synthetic tissues may add more to the array of option available for the reconstructive surgeons. Urethral tissue has been harvested from human cadaveric donor, converted to matrix graft enzymatically and use as graft for urethral reconstruction with no immunesuppression, no complication and satisfactory outcome. (Ribero-Filho et al, 2006) However, bioengineering and tissue culture are marking the future of urethral reconstruction because optimal tissues for urethral replacement will be produced by this technology. (Carson, 2006; MacAninch, 2005). Introduction of these tissues into clinical practice may actually be the beginning of a new era in urethral reconstruction.

9. Conclusion

Given the wide arrays of procedures available to urologist to reconstruct a strictured urethra, urologists should try to acquaint themselves with all the methods as a single technique cannot suffice for all stricture cases. More so, there are reasons why one technique can be chosen over another in each particular case. Where there are multiple options, I feel the experience of attending urologists should guide them in the choice of technique to treat each case.

10. References

Barbagli G, Palminteri E, Balo S, Vallasciani S, Mearini E, Constantini E, Mearini L, Zucchi A, Vivacqua C, & Porena M. (2004). Lichen sclerosis of the male genitalia and urethral stricture disease. *Urol Int,* 73, 1–5.

Brandes SB. (2008). Vascular anatomy of the genital skin and the urethra: Implications for urethral reconstruction. In: *Current Clinical Urology: Urethral Reconstructive Surgery,* SB Brandes, (Ed.) *153-164,* Humana Press, ISBN-978-1-588-29826-3, Totowa, NJ.

Buckley J & MacAninch J. (2007). Distal penile circular fascio-cutaneous flap for complex anterior urethral strictures. *BJU,* 100, 221-231.

Carney KJ & McAninch JW (2002) Penile circular fasciocutaneous flaps to reconstruct complex anterior urethral strictures. *Urol Clin N Am* 29:97–409.

Carson CC. (2006). Urethroplasty: a model for international progress in urology. *Contemp Urol.,* 18, 11.

Crew JP, Nargund V & Fellows GJ. (1996). Symptomatic urethral ball and Diverticulum complicating island flap urethroplasty. *Scand J Urol Nephro,* 30, 231-233.

Elliot SP & McAninch JW. (2008). Penile skin flap for urethral reconstruction, In: *Current Clinical Urology: Urethral Reconstructive Surgery,* SB Brandes, (Ed.) *153-164,* Humana Press, ISBN-978-1-588-29826-3, Totowa, NJ.

Finkelstein LH & Blatstein LM. (1991). Epilation of hair bearing urethral grafts using the neodymium:YAG surgical laser. *J Urol,* 146, 840-842.

Hinman Jr. F. The blood supply to preputial island flaps. (1991). *J Urol,* 145, 1232-1235.

Imamoglu MA, Kiper A, Tuygun C & Gucuk A. (2003). Results of TIPU on patients with primary and recurrent hypospadias. *J.Ankara Med.Sch.,* 25(4), 179-84.

Jordan GH & Rourke KF. (2005) The use of flaps in urethral reconstructive surgery. In: Reconstructive Urethral Surgery. Schreiter F & Jordan GH, (Eds.) 130-136, Springer, ISBN- 978-3-540-41226-7,

Kellner DS, Fracchia JA & Armenakas NA. (2004). Ventral onlay buccal mucosal grafts for anterior urethral strictures: long-term followup. *J Urol* 171: 726–729, 2004.

MacDonald MF & Santucci RA. (2005). Review and treatment algorithm of open surgical techniques for management of urethral strictures. *Urology,* 65, 9-15.

McAninch JW: (2005). Urethral reconstruction: a continuing challenge. *J Urol.,* 73, 7.

Mundy AR. Results and complications of urethroplasty and its future. (1993). *BJU,* 71, 322-325.

Mundy AR. (1995). The long term results of skin inlay urethroplasty. *BJU,* 75, 59-61.

Olajide AO, Salako AA, Aremu AA, Amogu KE, Olajide FO & Banjo OO. (2010). Complications of transverse distal penile island flap urethroplasty of complex anterior urethral stricture. *Urology Journal,* 7, 78-182.

Quartey JKM. (1987) One stage penile/preputial island flap urethroplasty for difficult posterior urethral stricture. *World J Urol,* 5, 37-40.

Ribeiro-Filho LA, Mitre AI, Sarkis AS, Guimaraes PE, Arap MA, Silva IA, et al. (2006). Human organ-specific acellular matrix grafting for severe urethral stenosis. *J Urol.,* 175: 161.

Rosen MA, Nash PA, Bruce J E, & McAninch J W. (1994). The actuarial success rate of surgical treatment of urethral strictures. *J Urol.,* 151, 360A, 529.

Sowande OA, Olajide AO, Salako AA, Olajide FO, Adejuyigbe O. Talabi AO. (2009). Experience with transverse preputial island flap for repair of hypospadias in Ile-Ife, Nigeria. African Journal of Paediatric Surgery, 6 (1), 40-43.

Santucci RA, Mario LA & McAninch JW. (2002). Anastomotic urethroplasty for bulbar urethral stricture: analysis of 168 patients. *J Urol* 167, 1715–1719.

Tung TA & Christopher MN. (2008). Techniques in tissue transfer: plastic surgery for the Urologist. In: *Current Clinical Urology: Urethral Reconstructive Surgery,* SB Brandes, (Ed.) *153-164,* Humana Press, ISBN-978-1-588-29826-3, Totowa, NJ.

11

The Use of Buccal Mucosa in Bulbar Stricture Repair: Morbidity and Functional Outcome

Frank Van der Aa, Kathy Vander Eeckt and Steven Joniau
Department of Urology, University Hospitals Leuven, Leuven
Belgium

1. Introduction

Urethral stricture disease is as old as mankind. In the old times urethral strictures were mainly associated with longstanding infectious disease (gonococcal urethritis) or trauma (Beard and Goodyear, 1948). Current stricture aetiology in the developed world is mainly iatrogenic, such as strictures after (traumatic) urethral catheterization or transurethral resection, and idiopathic (Fenton et al., 2005, Lumen et al., 2009). Besides the aetiology of strictures, also the armamentarium to treat them has evolved. Repeated dilatation or, in complicated cases, external urethrotomy or cystotomy were the only treatment options for centuries instead of leaving the disease on its natural evolution. Today, optic urethrotomy, anastomotic urethroplasty and substitution urethroplasty offer better functional results, better cosmesis and in the majority of patients a permanent solution to the disease.

Urethral strictures most frequently occur at the bulbar urethra (Lumen et al., 2009, Fenton et al., 2005, Meeks et al., 2009, Andrich and Mundy, 2008, Santucci et al., 2007). This is the part of the urethra that is surrounded by the corpus spongiosum and the bulbospongiosus muscle. When a bulbar stricture is encountered for the first time in a patient, a direct vision internal urethrotomy can be offered. This may be curative for short strictures in about half of the patients treated. Previous urethrotomy/dilatation or direct vision internal urethrotomy in longer strictures reduces success rates to almost zero (Pansadoro and Emiliozzi, 1996, Steenkamp et al., 1997). This does not mean that the patient cannot be managed this way, but the treatment is palliative in nature and repeat treatments or intermittent self catheterization will be mandatory to maintain patency.

When these patients want to be cured from their stricture disease, an operative approach has to be offered. It is probably better to offer this approach sooner than later. From a surgical point of view, less spongiofibrosis will be found and from an economical point of view, early surgery is probably more cost effective (Rourke and Jordan, 2005, Greenwell et al., 2004, Andrich and Mundy, 2008, Wright et al., 2006).

The operative approach can essentially be divided in anastomotic and substitution urethroplasties. In the first, a tension free, spatulated anastomosis is the key to success. This technique is generally advocated for shorter strictures that can be excised completely. It is assumed that results from end-to-end anastomotic urethroplasty are superior to substitution urethroplasty. This believe is partially based on intuition: excision of the diseased urethra and subsequent restoration of the continuity using healthy ends 'has to be better' then leaving the diseased urethra in place and augmenting it with another tissue. However, the evidence to support this believe is not solid (Meeks et al., 2009, Andrich et al., 2003). In a substitution urethroplasty, the urethral lumen calibre is restored using flaps (derived from scrotal or penile skin, tunica vaginalis,...) or grafts (skin, buccal mucosa, lingual mucosa, small intestinal submucosa,...) (Mangera et al.). This technique has become more widespread after the introduction of buccal mucosa as a free graft. Buccal mucosa offers a relatively resilient and easy to handle graft, rendering this surgery more accessible.

In the following chapter we will discuss the advantages and disadvantages of buccal mucosa free graft in the treatment of bulbar urethral stricture disease. We will not only focus on success as defined by absence of stricture recurrence but also on functional results and patient reported outcomes.

2. The rationale of using buccal mucosa free grafts in urethral stricture repair

For many years, oral mucosa has been used for reconstructing oral and maxillofacial defects, repairing the conjunctival mucosa of the eye, oral pharyngeal reconstructive surgery and reconstructing vaginal defects (Markiewicz et al., 2007). In 1941, Humby published the first report on the use of oral mucosa for urethroplastic repair, in which he used lingual mucosa graft (LMG) in a patient who had undergone previous unsuccessful hypospadias repair resulting in a fibrotic urethra and a penoscrotal fistula. It was not until 1992 when Burger et al (Burger et al., 1992) reintroduced oral mucosa as a graft source for urethroplastic procedures that the use of oral mucosa in reconstructive urology gained widespread use. A month after the report by Burger et al was published, Dessanti et al (Dessanti et al., 1992) reported on 8 combined bladder mucosa and autologous LMGs for hypospadias repair.

Although there has been some dispute among authors as to who actually reintroduced the oral mucosa graft into contemporary reconstructive urology practice, we credit Burger and Dessanti et al for their groundbreaking work.

The two most common sites of oral mucosa harvest for urethral repair are the labial alveolar and the buccal mucosa. Oral mucosa has a thick nonkeratinized stratified squamous avascular epithelium and a slightly vascular underlying lamina propria (Duckett et al., 1995). Oral mucosa is exceptionally appropriate for urethral substitution because it is architecturally similar to the stratified squamous epithelium of the penile and glandular urethra. Because of sufficient graft surface, oral mucosa is easy to harvest. Frequently exposed to compression, stretching and shearing forces, the oral mucosa is highly resilient. Blood vessels and nerve fibres from the submucosa infiltrate into the lamina propria and provide a mechanism for angiogenesis and revascularization of the tissue when grafting (Duckett et al., 1995). Oral mucosa is resistant to infection because the oral epithelial cells are infused with polymicrobial intracellular and extracellular flora (Rudney and Chen, 2006), the mucosal epithelial cells limit microflora by a specialized immune system (MALT) and the well-defatted lamina propria of the oral mucosa graft is a secondary barrier preventing microorganisms from entering adjacent tissue layers (Walker, 2004).

3. Functional outcome of bulbar urethral stricture repair using buccal mucosa

The functional outcome of urethral surgery is often reported in terms of urethral patency only. Although this is an obvious and essential outcome parameter, since this is the reason for surgery in the first place, it is also important to look into continence, erectile and ejaculatory function, post void dribbling and patient satisfaction in general. In other words: both the urologist and the patient should be satisfied with the obtained result.

3.1 Success of urethral repair

Bulbar urethral stricture repair using buccal mucosa provides high success rates. Depending on the definition of failure, the length of follow up and the technique used to augment the urethra, success rates vary between 65,8% and 100% with an average of more than 80% (Mangera et al.). Failure can be defined as a certain Q_{max} value using uroflowmetry. This value is easily obtainable, but is a reflection of different functional aspects such as urethral diameter, detrusor contraction and abdominal straining. The diameter of the urethra has to decrease very substantially (to less than 10 french) before a clear impact on flow rate is noticed (Smith, 1966). Abdominal straining can mask low urethral diameters. Therefore this is a variable and relative late sign for failure. Patient reported outcome parameters, such as symptom scores or the need for instrumentation can be used as parameters of failure. One can also expect late diagnosis of recurrence using these methods for exactly the same reasons. Urethrography is advocated by some authors to follow up urethral stricture repair in a more objective way. Others disagree, because images are not always easy to interpret, and argue that endoscopic evaluation gives a clear and objective definition of patency after repair. It is sure that endoscopic evaluation is the only certain outcome parameter. We also promote endoscopic evaluation in the follow up of urethral stricture repair. In retrospective series however it is not always possible to obtain these data. Future studies that are designed in a prospective way should take this into account. It is on the other hand not always easy to perform an invasive investigation on a patient when he reports to be satisfied.

Longer follow up times result in less favourable outcome. Barbagli et al. showed that even after longer time, the number of stricture recurrences rose steadily (Barbagli et al., 1997). It is not clear whether a plateau phase of the recurrence curve is encountered at a certain time point. Follow up times of less than one year might overestimate the success rate of a technique.

Several techniques of bulbar urethral stricture repair using buccal mucosa have been reported in literature. The traditional technique of ventral onlay urethroplasty has reported success rates from 80 to 100% (Meneghini et al., 2001, Morey and McAninch, 1996, Barbagli et al., 2008b, Wessells and McAninch, 1996). One report of 7 patients only had a success rate of 43% (Berger et al., 2005). In a recent meta analysis an overall success rate for ventral onlay urethroplasty of 88,84% with an average follow up of 34,3 months in 563 patients was calculated from the existing literature (Mangera et al., 2011).

Since the first description in 1996 of the dorsal onlay urethroplasty by Barbagli et al., this technique has gained widespread acceptation by urethral surgeons worldwide (Barbagli et al., 1996). Reported success rates are very high and vary from 77,3% to 100% (Barbagli et al., 2008b, Barbagli et al., 2006, Joseph et al., 2002). Again, a pooled analysis of all published data on dorsal onlay urethroplasty calculated an overall success rate of 88,37% for 943 patients treated with an average follow up of 42,2 months (Mangera et al., 2011). In our own series of 61 patients, we encountered an estimated failure free rate of 90,2% with an average follow up of 25,3 months (Vander Eeckt and Joniau, 2010a).

Other, less frequently used techniques, such as lateral onlay urethroplasty, two sided urethroplasty, augmented anastomosis and the Asopa technique have been reported as well. The results of these techniques are comparable to the above mentioned, more classical techniques. The number of patients treated with these techniques is rather small and the description comes from selected centres (Barbagli et al., 2005, Barbagli et al., 2008b, Pisapati et al., 2009, Palminteri et al.). In augmented anastomotic urethroplasty, reported success rates can attain more than 90% after more than 2 years of follow up in a complex patient population (Guralnick and Webster, 2001).

In large series of end-to-end urethroplasty, comparable outcome is reached with success rates reaching around 90% after 26 and more than 60 months follow up respectively (Gupta et al., 2009, Barbagli et al., 2007).

In our patient population of 103 patients, 61 underwent bulbar stricture repair with a dorsal onlay buccal mucosa graft and 42 underwent an end-to-end repair. The re-stricture rate of buccal mucosa graft repair was not significantly different from end-to-end repair(Vander Eeckt et al., 2010). Preoperative strictures in the former group were significantly longer and a significantly higher number of patients in that group had undergone previous reconstructive urethral surgery. This makes a direct comparison of results impossible, but indicates that dorsal onlay urethroplasty is certainly not inferior to end-to-end repair in our hands.

In general, substitution urethroplasty with buccal mucosa can attain very high success rates which are comparable to anastomotic urethroplasty, even in the longer strictures. Whenever a traction free anastomosis cannot be achieved, one should not hesitate to use free graft repair.

3.2 Post void dribbling

Post void dribbling is a known complication of substitution urethroplasty. This is mainly caused by splitting the bulbourethral muscle longitudinally. The augmentation of the urethra creates a somewhat dilated and atonic part where urine can reside for a while and dribble out in the minutes after micturition. Furthermore, the dissection, transsection or opening of the urethra can create deficient closing mechanisms. The problem is reported to be worse after ventral onlay urethroplasty (up to 1/3 of patients), attributed to increased dilatation of the graft as compared to dorsal onlay urethroplasty (around 1/10 patients) (Fransis et al., 2009, Joseph et al., 2002, Bhandari et al., 2001). These differences are not reproduced by all authors. We even found similar post void dribbling incidences in end-to-end anastomosis as compared to buccal mucosa dorsal onlay urethroplasty when we actively asked patients whether they had post void dribbling (Vander Eeckt and Joniau, 2010a). Although it is an "innocent" symptom, it can lower quality of life. Patients should be counselled preoperatively about this surgical side effect and should be taught how to empty the anterior urethra after micturition. Muscle and nerve sparing techniques might eliminate these side effects of urethral surgery, although only occasional reports have been published to date (Barbagli et al., 2008a).

3.3 Urinary incontinence

In general, urinary continence is not affected by urethroplasty. In certain subgroups of patients however, this might be an expected and invalidating side effect of urethral surgery. Patients that underwent previous prostatic surgery are at specific risk for this invalidating side effect. Also a history of radiotherapy might predispose for this condition. Meeks et al. recently reported on 30 patients with radiation induced strictures. Exactly half (15/30) of the patients developed incontinence. In the minority of patients (3/30) this was a transient phenomenon, but in 12/30 (40%) of patients this incontinence was long lasting. In the end

4/30 (13%) patients finally required an artificial urinary sphincter implant to restore continence (Meeks et al., 2011). This is in accordance with sporadic clinical experience of severe incontinence after complex urological history. It is not always easy to predict this functional outcome, but patients have to be counselled for this possibility since it may have a tremendous impact on the quality of life. Furthermore, bulbar placement of an artificial urinary sphincter might not always be possible, due to the previous urethral surgery.

3.4 Erectile and ejaculatory dysfunction

As illustrated above, the evidence in favor of surgical treatment of urethral stricture disease has accumulated. This trend has caused more concerns about postoperative complications like erectile dysfunction and ejaculatory dysfunction after urethral surgery.

The theoretical risk of **erectile dysfunction** comes due to the close relationship of the cavernous nerves with the proximal urethra when they emerge from the pelvic floor. Nerve fibers emerge from the anterior foramina of S2-S4 and join the fibers from the hypogastric nerve to form the pelvic plexus; The most caudal fibers of the plexus travel along the posterolateral side of the prostate and innervate the corpora of the penis. This is the *cavernous nerve* responsible for penile erection (Lue et al., 1984). The carvernous nerves form several bundles on each side of the urethra at 3 and 9 o'clock positions. At the proximal bulbar urethra some fibers penetrate the tunica albuginea of the corpus spongiosum to innervate the vasculature and erectile tissues of the corpus spongiosum and glans penis. The rest of the fibers remain outside the corpus spongiosum and ascend gradually to the 1 and 11 o'clock positions at the level in which the crura of the corpora cavernosa converge to the midline (Lue et al., 1984).

Yucel et al (Yucel and Baskin, 2003) have shown that the *perineal nerve* may also have a role in erectile dysfunction. Intimate communications ware found between the cavernous, dorsal and perineal nerve fibers and at these communications, the dorsal and perineal nerve (they do not innervate the erectile bodies directly) contain nitric oxide synthase, responsible for production of NO. This suggests that they play a role in vasodilatation of penile arteries.

Normal ejaculation requires 3 steps including ejaculate emission into the urethra by alfa-adrenergic contractions of the prostate, seminal vesicles and vas deferens, bladder neck contraction to prevent retrograde ejaculation and finally semen expulsion from the urethra by bulbocavernous and ischiocavernous muscle contraction. Disruption in one of those steps alter normal ejaculation. The *perineal nerve* (S3-S4) is critical for the bulbocavernous reflex contraction and sensory function of the perineum. After the pudendal nerve leaves the pudendal canal it gives rise to the perineal nerve branches. Perineal nerves travel along the ischiocavernous and bulbospongiosus muscles. Fine nerve fibers arise from the lateral trunk and travel to the junction of the two muscle bellies in the midline to pierce into the midline and send branches to the corpus spongiosum.

The *dorsal nerve* of the penis is the deepest division of the pudendal nerve. It gives branches to the corpus cavernosum of the penis and goes on to the dorsum of the penis and ends in the glans penis; It innervates the skin of the penis. (Yang and Bradley, 1999)

Previous studies have focused more on stricture recurrence and incontinence and only a small part of the reports discussed erectile dysfunction. More recent reports are starting to evaluate potency after urethral stricture repair.

Mundy et al (Mundy, 1993) was the first to comment on ED after urethroplasty, reporting a permanent ED rate of 5% after anastomotic repairs and 0,9% after graft urethroplasty. Coursey et al (Coursey et al., 2001) reported in 2001 a retrospective analysis of 250 men after urethroplasty. At a mean follow-up of 36 months 26,8% was not satisfied with the erection after anastomotic urethroplasty and 19,2% after buccal mucosa graft. Anger et al (Anger et al., 2007) were the first to publish a prospective study of 25 men undergoing bulbar urethroplasty using the IIEF questionnaire. They found that urethroplasty had no significant effect on erectile function. Also Barbagli et al (Barbagli et al., 2007) reported no impotence in a review of 153 patients with an average age of 39 years who underwent bulbar end-to-end anastomosis. Erickson et al (Erickson et al., 2010) published a prospective study of 25 men using the IIEF score. Although there was no statistically significant difference between the ED after anastomotic (50%) versus buccal mucosa graft urethroplasty (26%), there was a trend towards a higher rate of erectile dysfunction after anastomotic repair. Xie et al (Xie et al., 2009) published prospective study of 152 patients after urethroplasty. Postoperatively 69,6% patients had an increased erectile dysfunction. However, there was a rebound of IIEF-5 score at 6 months post-operatively, but this was only observed in men younger than 40 years. End-to-end anastomosis was associated with an lower IIEF-5 score.

In our experience, we performed a retrospective comparison between a bulbar urethroplasty were the urethra was transected (anastomotic and buccal mucosa roof strip augmented urethroplasty) and a bulbar urethroplasty were the urethra was not transected (dorsal inlay buccal mucosa urethroplasty) (Vander Eeckt and Joniau, 2010b). We saw a significant lower IIEF-5 postoperatively after transecting the urethra (P=0,0017). After urethroplasty were the urethra was not transected the IIEF-5 was not significantly lower (P=0,21).

All presented studies have limitations; They have a limited follow-up, small population and not all studies are prospective. The largest limitation is the lack of a validated questionnaire, specifically created for erectile function after urethroplasty; changes in angle of the erection, length of the penis, swelling of the glans or changes in penile sensitivity.

Despite these limitations, a trend toward increased erectile dysfunction after anastomotic bulbar urethroplasty compared with buccal mucosa graft urethroplasty is seen. The exact reason is not yet known but there are some hypotheses:

i. Extensive dissection and mobilization at the level of the convergence of the corpora cavernosa in anastomotic urethroplasty may damage the cavernous nerves at that level. Sometimes even splitting of the corpora cavernosa is necessary to avoid traction on the anastomosis;
ii. In order to expose the underlying corpus spongiosum, splitting of the bulbospongiosus muscle is necessary. This is frequently accompanied by a disruption of the perineal nerves. In order to avoid this, Barbagli et al (Barbagli et al., 2008a) described a muscle and nerve sparing bulbar urethroplasty using buccal mucosa. Unfortunately this is not possible for anastomotic urethroplasty. Therefore, damaging the perineal nerves occur more in anastomotic urethroplasty than in buccal mucosa urethroplasty. As noted in "part one" the perineal nerve is not only responsible for ejaculation but has probably a role in erectile function. (Yucel and Baskin, 2003)
iii. At the proximal bulbar urethra, some cavernous fibers penetrate the tunica albuginea of the corpus spongiosum to innervate the vasculature and erectile tissues of the corpus spongiosum and glans penis. Transection of the urethra during a anastomotic urethroplasty not only implies suturing this vasculature but also the nerve fibers close to and in the corpus spongiosum.

Ejaculatory function following urethroplasty has been studied considerably less than erectile dysfunction.

The effect of urethroplasty on ejaculation has not yet been proved but there are some hypotheses. On the one hand obstruction relief may allow semen to travel with less impedance through the urethra, on the other hand splitting through the bulbocavernous muscle and dissecting around the urethra might harm neurovascular integrity.

Author	Number of pts (FU in months	End-to-end	Buccal mucosa
Mundy et al. BJU (Mundy, 1993)	200 (?) (? M)	5%	0.9% ("patch")
Coursey et al. J Urol (Coursey et al., 2001)	82 (36 m)	26.8%	19.2%
Anger et al. J Urol (Anger et al., 2007)	25 (6.2 m)	Global: no difference in preop and postoperative ED 1/8 end-to-end: wel postop ED	
Barbagli et al. J Urol (Barbagli et al., 2007)	60 (68 m)	Global: no difference in preop and postoperative ED 31.6% 'neurovascular disorder'	
Erickson et al J Urol (Erickson et al., 2010)	35 (6,2m)	50%	26%
Our experience (Vander Eeckt and Joniau, 2010a)	48 (25 m)	26.1%	15.4%

Table 1. Erectile dysfunction after urethroplasty

Barbagli et al (Barbagli et al., 2007) reported ejaculatory dysfunction in a study of 60 patients after anastomotic urethroplasty but not after the use of buccal mucosa. There were 14 patients (23.3%) who experienced ejaculatory dysfunction, 1 (1.6%) a cold glans during erection, 7 (11.6%) a glans that was neither full nor swollen during erection and 11 (18.3%) had decreased glans sensitivity. No patients complained of penile chordee or impotence. Erickson et al (Erickson et al., 2010) is the first who presented a prospective analysis of ejaculatory function after anterior urethral reconstruction using the Male Sexual Health Questionnaire. A total of 43 men were included, the overall ejaculatory score did not change postoperatively at a mean follow-up of 8,1 months but men with a poor preoperative function had a significant improvement. Postoperative function was stable in 70%, improved in 19% and worsened in 11%. There was no significant difference between the penile and bulbar urethroplasty. Unfortunately, he made no difference between anastomotic or buccal mucosa graft urethroplasty.

In our experience, we compared the ejaculatory function between anastomotic urethroplasty and a urethroplasty with buccal mucosa. The remembered ejaculatory dysfunction was around 33-38%. Postoperatively patients after anastomotic urethroplasty had more ejaculatory dysfunction (45%) when compared to buccal mucosa urethroplasty (30,7%) (P=0,033) (Vander Eeckt and Joniau, 2010a).

3.5 Donor site morbidity

Before harvesting buccal mucosa, the surgeon must be aware of the anatomy of the buccal cavity. The buccal cavity is innervated by the long buccal nerve and by the second division of the trigeminal nerve. Additionally, there is sensory innervation from the facial nerve. The blood supply originates from a branch of the buccal artery, a branch of the maxillary artery and a branch of the superficial temporal artery. The surgeon must be aware of the Stenson's' duct that originates of the parotid gland. The orifice is visible by a papilla on the mucosa. Underneath the mucosa lies the buccinator muscle. Failure to operate away of these structures may result in damage to the parotid duct with postoperative symptoms of the salivary obstruction; limitation of oral opening because of scarring and contracture; intra-operative hemorrhage; diminished ability to eat and drink; postoperative infection; pain, swelling, and injury to the long buccal or mental nerves with subsequent paresthesia or anesthesia of the cheek.

Nasal endotracheal intubation is preferred to facilitate to the oral cavity, although oral endotracheal intubation is possible. The patient is positioned for a two-team approach to reduce the patient's time in the lithotomy position. Two separate surgical tables are prepared to minimize contamination of the oral wound to the urologic wound. After measuring the intraoperative urethral defect, the extent and shape of the buccal mucosa graft must be marked by a surgical pen. The surgeon must be aware that the graft shrinks up to 20% of their original size. Care must be taken to stay at least 8 mm below the papilla of stenson's duct and at least 1cm behind the vermillion border. Local anesthetic is injected to decrease the bleeding, help elevate and hydro-dissect the buccal mucosa from the underlying soft tissue. Blunt and sharp dissection with a metzenbaum scissors may be used. The intraoral wound can be closed or left open. Then the harvest tissue is prepared by removing any muscle or adipose tissue. The prepared graft is kept in a 0,9% saline solution until used for reconstruction.

Although the buccal mucosa is the graft of choice in many circumstances, only few data about the morbidity of the harvest site are available (table 2).

Early complications such as **bleeding** did not occur in the first reports (Kamp et al., 2005, Eppley, 1997, Burger et al., 1992, Tolstunov et al., 1997, Morey and McAninch, 1996, Wood et al., 2004). More recent studies report postoperative bleeding between 2,5 and 21%. In most of the patients it is self-limiting but some patients need immediate surgical revision of the harvesting site (Barbagli et al., 2010, Fabbroni et al., 2005).

After buccal mucosa harvest patient could expect some **pain and discomfort**. Abdel-Galil et al (Abdel-Galil et al., 2009) reported a prospective study of 24 patients using a visual analogue pain scale of the harvest site and the perineum the first 48h. This shows that the perineal pain was significantly higher than the pain at the donor site ($p< 0,001$). Almost all patients have immediate postoperative pain but this usually resolves within 3 weeks postoperatively (Tolstunov et al., 1997, Jang et al., 2005, Kamp et al., 2005, Dublin and Stewart, 2004). Two studies compared the postoperative morbidity after harvesting of the lip versus buccal mucosa. Harvesting from the lip resulted in significantly greater long-term morbidity, this seems due to the long-lasting neuropathy of the mental nerve (Kamp et al., 2005, Jang et al., 2005). Some studies compared closure versus non closure of the buccal mucosa graft harvest site (Wood et al., 2004, Muruganandam et al., 2009). Pain appears worse in the immediate post operative period with suturing of the harvest site. It may be best to leave the buccal mucosa harvest site unsutured.

Patients who have had a BMG harvest can also expect to have a limited range of **jaw opening** (Dublin and Stewart, 2004, Tolstunov et al., 1997). Tolstunov et al (Tolstunov et al., 1997) measured the preoperative mouth opening preoperatively, and then after 1week, 2-3-6 weeks and 6 months. Almost all patient had difficulties with mouth opening the first week postoperatively, but all patients returned to their preoperative mouth opening; Recent studies did report persistent difficulties in jaw opening between 1,7 and 32%. Jang et al compared the morbidity between labial and buccal mucosa. Contractures were more common in patients whose grafts were harvested from the cheek, presumably from the increased incidence of closure of the harvest site. Because of this, it is better to leave the harvest site open.

After reconstruction of extensive strictures using large grafts, patients can expect more **neurosensory deficit** than after a small graft. These deficits usually last up to 1 month. Some studies reported a persistent oral numbness between 3,77 and 40% (Wood et al., 2004, Dublin and Stewart, 2004, Kamp et al., 2005, Jang et al., 2005, Castagnetti et al., 2008). LMG harvest is associated with a greater chance of mental nerve damage then BMG harvest because of the anatomy of the mental nerve. Jang et al (Jang et al., 2005) published a study were he compared morbidity after labial and the buccal harvest sites. BMG harvest was associated with less postoperative discomfort, less neurosensory defect.

No cases with permanent damage to the parotid duct with resulting salivary flow obstruction have been reported. Damaging the salivary glands, mild temporary decrease of **salivary flow** is reported. In most of the patients this resolved in the first week (Tolstunov et al., 1997), although in 2,6%-11% of the patients a slight or moderate dry mouth persisted (Wood et al., 2004, Castagnetti et al., 2008). Comparing morbidity after labial and the buccal harvest sites, Jang et al (Jang et al., 2005) reported less salivary flow after Labial mucosa graft than BMG. Less salivary flow would be expected because the labial mucosa contains more minor salivary gland tissue than the buccal mucosa (Tolstunov et al., 1997). It is nearly impossible to harvest a labial mucosa graft without interfering with the salivary secretion.

Some studies assessed the **quality of life** after harvesting oral mucosa. A recent large study of 350 patients by Barbagli et al. (Barbagli et al., 2010), assessed the QOL. In response to the question, "would you undergo buccal mucosa graft harvesting using this technique again", only 2% said 'no' to the question. Dublin et al (Dublin and Stewart, 2004) asked a similar question and reported that 3% of the patients were dissatisfied and 23% had mixed feelings. Comparing LMG and BMG harvest patients after LMG harvest (50%) seemed less satisfied than those after BMG harvest (8,3%). This was not confirmed in the study of Jang et al, probably because their QOL of life assessment reflected more the outcome of the reconstructive surgery than the morbidity of the harvest site.

In our experience early complications are rather frequent. We performed a retrospective analysis of 91 patients with a in-house developed questionnaire. During the first two weeks after surgery, up to 14,3 % of the patients had pain and 45.5% had problems with eating solid food, 32.1% had jaw opening impairment and 26,8% had oral numbness. After a median follow-up of 31,4 months, oral numbness remains the most important complaint (up to 20,4%), while 2,3% had problems with contractures (Vander Eeckt and Joniau, 2010c). These results are comparable with the result mentioned in the literature. Other complaints were infrequent after six months.

All studies about the morbidity of buccal mucosa graft taking, have limitations. First, some complaints like pain or neurosensory deficit are difficult to evaluate objectively. Second, although most of the questionnaires are reliable, all studies are limited because of the absence of validated instruments to evaluate pain, the harvest site morbidity, and typical quality of life changes. Third, most of the studies have small patient numbers and limited follow-up. The development of validated questionnaires and large prospective studies are needed to assess the morbidity after oral mucosa graft taking.

Author(s)	year	FU months	short term (%)		long term complications (%)			
			Pain	Hematoma	numbness	jaw opening	pain	Less salivary flow
Burger et al (Burger et al., 1992)	1992		no complications					
Morey et al (Morey and McAninch, 1996)	1996	18	no complications					
Tolstunov et al (Tolstunov et al., 1997)	1997	3		0	0	0		0
Eppley et al (Eppley, 1997)	1997		0	0			0	
Dublin et al (Dublin and Stewart, 2004)	2004	13.6	64	0	16	32	0	
Wood et al (Wood et al., 2004)	2004		83		26	9		11
Kamp et al (Kamp et al., 2005)	2005	12.5	100	0	25		16	
Fabbroni et al(Fabbroni et al., 2005)	2005	3		4.3		4		
Jang et al (Jang et al., 2005)	2005	12	4.67	2.5	40	20	0	
Castagnetti et al (Castagnetti et al., 2008)	2008	7.6y		21	28	2.6		2.6
Barbagli et al (Barbagli et al., 2010)	2010	6	3.7	4.3	3.77	1.7		2.9

Table 2. Reports on long term morbidity associated with buccal mucosa harvest site

4. Conclusions

Bulbar urethral stricture disease is a curable disease. Palliative treatment such as recurrent dilatations or urethrotomies should only be offered to very selected patients with high comorbidities or who refuse surgery. Stricture repair using buccal mucosa offers a technique that has proven to be effective and reproducible with high stricture-free rates.

However, buccal mucosa graft harvesting is not without morbidity and when reporting the success of urethral surgery, one should also take into account surgical morbidity, functional results and patient satisfaction.

At the functional level, *post void dribbling* will occur relatively frequently after stricture repair. When patients are counselled preoperatively for this side effect and when they are learned to empty their urethra manually, this side-effect becomes manageable and accepted by most patients.

Urinary incontinence is a rare but devastating complication of stricture repair in a selected group of patients. In these difficult cases, one should only embark in stricture repair after careful counselling and after discussing potential future therapies to treat incontinence.

The consequences of urethral stricture repair on *sexual function* are not entirely clear.

As shown above, studies on ejaculatory dysfunction are few in numbers and small in study size. More studies are needed, but this is not easy because of the lack of standardization in pre- and postoperative investigations and the absence of validated questionnaires including measurement of bulbocavernous muscle contractile potential, ejaculation latency time, ejaculate volume... Similarly, typical changes in erection after urethral surgery ('cold glans syndrome', sensory deficit at glans level, chordate, curvature, shortening of penile length) are not captured by commonly accepted erectile function scales (like IIEF-score). Nevertheless, compared to anastomotic repair, buccal mucosa graft urethroplasty seems to cause less erectile dysfunction.

Notwithstanding these shortcomings in the literature, this chapter has clearly shown that the use of oral mucosa free grafts leads to excellent stricture-free rates. Furthermore, functional results (more specifically, erectile function results) surpass those of other reconstructive approaches, while graft site morbidity is very acceptable in the short term and almost negligible in the long term.

5. References

Abdel-Galil, K., Eardley, I. & Loukota, R. (2009) Buccal mucosal grafts for urethroplasty: comparison of postoperative oral and perineal morbidity. *Ann R Coll Surg Engl*, 91, 116-7.

Andrich, D. E., Dunglison, N., Greenwell, T. J. & Mundy, A. R. (2003) The long-term results of urethroplasty. *J Urol*, 170, 90-2.

Andrich, D. E. & Mundy, A. R. (2008) What is the best technique for urethroplasty? *Eur Urol*, 54, 1031-41.

Anger, J. T., Sherman, N. D. & Webster, G. D. (2007) The effect of bulbar urethroplasty on erectile function. *J Urol*, 178, 1009-11; discussion 1011.

Barbagli, G., De Angelis, M., Romano, G. & Lazzeri, M. (2007) Long-term followup of bulbar end-to-end anastomosis: a retrospective analysis of 153 patients in a single center experience. *J Urol*, 178, 2470-3.

Barbagli, G., De Stefani, S., Annino, F., De Carne, C. & Bianchi, G. (2008a) Muscle- and nerve-sparing bulbar urethroplasty: a new technique. *Eur Urol*, 54, 335-43.

Barbagli, G., De Stefani, S., Sighinolfi, M. C., Annino, F., Micali, S. & BIANCHI, G. (2006) Bulbar urethroplasty with dorsal onlay buccal mucosal graft and fibrin glue. *Eur Urol*, 50, 467-74.

Barbagli, G., Guazzoni, G. & Lazzeri, M. (2008b) One-stage bulbar urethroplasty: retrospective analysis of the results in 375 patients. *Eur Urol*, 53, 828-33.

Barbagli, G., Palminteri, E., Bartoletti, R., Selli, C. & Rizzo, M. (1997) Long-term results of anterior and posterior urethroplasty with actuarial evaluation of the success rates. *J Urol*, 158, 1380-2.

Barbagli, G., Palminteri, E., Guazzoni, G., Montorsi, F., Turini, D. & Lazzeri, M. (2005) Bulbar urethroplasty using buccal mucosa grafts placed on the ventral, dorsal or lateral surface of the urethra: are results affected by the surgical technique? *J Urol*, 174, 955-7; discussion 957-8.

Barbagli, G., Selli, C., Tosto, A. & Palminteri, E. (1996) Dorsal free graft urethroplasty. *J Urol*, 155, 123-6.

Barbagli, G., Vallasciani, S., Romano, G., Fabbri, F., Guazzoni, G. & Lazzeri, M. (2010) Morbidity of oral mucosa graft harvesting from a single cheek. *Eur Urol*, 58, 33-41.

Beard, D. E. & Goodyear, W. E. (1948) Urethral stricture; a pathological study. *J Urol*, 59, 619-26.

Berger, A. P., Deibl, M., Bartsch, G., Steiner, H., Varkarakis, J. & Gozzi, C. (2005) A comparison of one-stage procedures for post-traumatic urethral stricture repair. *BJU Int*, 95, 1299-302.

Bhandari, M., Dubey, D. & Verma, B. S. (2001) Dorsal or ventral placement of the preputial/penile skin onlay flap for anterior urethral strictures: does it make a difference? *BJU Int*, 88, 39-43.

Burger, R. A., Muller, S. C., El-Damanhoury, H., Tschakaloff, A., Riedmiller, H. & Hohenfellner, R. (1992) The buccal mucosal graft for urethral reconstruction: a preliminary report. *J Urol*, 147, 662-4.

Castagnetti, M., Ghirardo, V., Capizzi, A., Andretta, M. & Rigamonti, W. (2008) Donor site outcome after oral mucosa harvest for urethroplasty in children and adults. *J Urol*, 180, 2624-8.

Coursey, J. W., Morey, A. F., Mcaninch, J. W., Summerton, D. J., Secrest, C., White, P., Miller, K., Pieczonka, C., Hochberg, D. & Armenakas, N. (2001) Erectile function after anterior urethroplasty. *J Urol*, 166, 2273-6.

Dessanti, A., Rigamonti, W., Merulla, V., Falchetti, D. & Caccia, G. (1992) Autologous buccal mucosa graft for hypospadias repair: an initial report. *J Urol*, 147, 1081-3; discussion 1083-4.

Dublin, N. & Stewart, L. H. (2004) Oral complications after buccal mucosal graft harvest for urethroplasty. *BJU Int*, 94, 867-9.

Duckett, J. W., Coplen, D., Ewalt, D. & Baskin, L. S. (1995) Buccal mucosal urethral replacement. *The Journal of urology*, 153, 1660-3.

Eppley, B. L. (1997) A simplified technique for harvesting large buccal mucosal grafts. *J Oral Maxillofac Surg*, 55, 891-2.

Erickson, B. A., Granieri, M. A., Meeks, J. J., Cashy, J. P. & Gonzalez, C. M. (2010). Prospective analysis of erectile dysfunction after anterior urethroplasty: incidence and recovery of function. *J Urol*, 183, 657-61.

Fabbroni, G., Loukota, R. A. & Eardley, I. (2005) Buccal mucosal grafts for urethroplasty: surgical technique and morbidity. *Br J Oral Maxillofac Surg*, 43, 320-3.

Fenton, A. S., Morey, A. F., Aviles, R. & Garcia, C. R. (2005) Anterior urethral strictures: etiology and characteristics. *Urology*, 65, 1055-8.

Fransis, K., Vander Eeckt, K., Van Poppel, H. & Joniau, S. (2009) Results of buccal mucosa grafts for repairing long bulbar urethral strictures. *BJU Int*.

Greenwell, T. J., Castle, C., Andrich, D. E., Macdonald, J. T., Nicol, D. L. & Mundy, A. R. (2004) Repeat urethrotomy and dilation for the treatment of urethral stricture are neither clinically effective nor cost-effective. *J Urol*, 172, 275-7.

Gupta, N. P., Mishra, S., Dogra, P. N., Hemal, A. K., Seth, A. & Kumar, R. (2009) Outcome of end-to-end urethroplasty: single-center experience. *Urol Int*, 82, 179-82.

Guralnick, M. L. & Webster, G. D. (2001) The augmented anastomotic urethroplasty: indications and outcome in 29 patients. *J Urol*, 165, 1496-501.

Jang, T. L., Erickson, B., Medendorp, A. & Gonzalez, C. M. (2005) Comparison of donor site intraoral morbidity after mucosal graft harvesting for urethral reconstruction. *Urology*, 66, 716-20.

Joseph, J. V., Andrich, D. E., Leach, C. J. & Mundy, A. R. (2002) Urethroplasty for refractory anterior urethral stricture. *J Urol*, 167, 127-9.

Kamp, S., Knoll, T., Osman, M., Hacker, A., Michel, M. S. & Alken, P. (2005) Donor-site morbidity in buccal mucosa urethroplasty: lower lip or inner cheek? *BJU Int,* 96, 619-23.

Lue, T. F., Zeineh, S. J., Schmidt, R. A. & Tanagho, E. A. (1984) Neuroanatomy Of penile erection: its relevance to iatrogenic impotence. *J Urol,* 131, 273-80.

Lumen, N., Hoebeke, P., Willemsen, P., De Troyer, B., Pieters, R. & Oosterlinck, W. (2009) Etiology of urethral stricture disease in the 21st century. *J Urol,* 182, 983-7.

Mangera, A., Patterson, J. M. & Chapple, C. R. A (2011) Systematic Review of Graft Augmentation Urethroplasty Techniques for the Treatment of Anterior Urethral Strictures. *Eur Urol,* 59, 797-814.

Markiewicz, M. R., Lukose, M. A., Margarone, J. E., 3rd, Barbagli, G., Miller, K. S. & Chuang, S. K. (2007) The oral mucosa graft: a systematic review. *J Urol,* 178, 387-94.

Meeks, J. J., Brandes, S. B., Morey, A. F., Thom, M., Mehdiratta, N., Valadez, C., Granieri, M. A. & Gonzalez, C. M. (2011) Urethroplasty for Radiotherapy Induced Bulbomembranous Strictures: A Multi-Institutional Experience. *J Urol,* 185(5),1761-5.

Meeks, J. J., Erickson, B. A., Granieri, M. A. & Gonzalez, C. M. (2009) Stricture recurrence after urethroplasty: a systematic review. *J Urol,* 182, 1266-70.

Meneghini, A., Cacciola, A., Cavarretta, L., Abatangelo, G., Ferrarrese, P. & Tasca, A. (2001) Bulbar urethral stricture repair with buccal mucosa graft urethroplasty. *Eur Urol,* 39, 264-7.

Morey, A. F. & Mcaninch, J. W. (1996) When and how to use buccal mucosal grafts in adult bulbar urethroplasty. *Urology,* 48, 194-8.

Mundy, A. R. (1993) Results and complications of urethroplasty and its future. *Br J Urol,* 71, 322-5.

Muruganandam, K., Dubey, D., Gulia, A. K., Mandhani, A., Srivastava, A., Kapoor, R. & Kumar, A. (2009) Closure versus nonclosure of buccal mucosal graft harvest site: A prospective randomized study on post operative morbidity. *Indian J Urol,* 25, 72-5.

Palminteri, E., Berdondini, E., Shokeir, A. A., Iannotta, L., Gentile, V. & Sciarra, A. Two-Sided Bulbar Urethroplasty Using Dorsal Plus Ventral Oral Graft: Urinary and Sexual Outcomes of a New Technique. *J Urol.*

Pansadoro, V. & Emiliozzi, P. (1996) Internal urethrotomy in the management of anterior urethral strictures: long-term followup. *J Urol,* 156, 73-5.

Pisapati, V. L., Paturi, S., Bethu, S., Jada, S., Chilumu, R., Devraj, R., Reddy, B. & Sriramoju, V. (2009) Dorsal buccal mucosal graft urethroplasty for anterior urethral stricture by Asopa technique. *Eur Urol,* 56, 201-5.

Rourke, K. F. & Jordan, G. H. (2005) Primary urethral reconstruction: the cost minimized approach to the bulbous urethral stricture. *J Urol,* 173, 1206-10.

Rudney, J. D. & Chen, R. (2006) The vital status of human buccal epithelial cells and the bacteria associated with them. *Arch Oral Biol,* 51, 291-8.

Santucci, R. A., Joyce, G. F. & Wise, M. (2007) Male urethral stricture disease. *J Urol,* 177, 1667-74.

Smith, J. C. (1966) The measurement and significance of the urinary flow rate. *Br J Urol,* 38, 701-6.

Steenkamp, J. W., Heyns, C. F. & De Kock, M. L. (1997) Internal urethrotomy versus dilation as treatment for male urethral strictures: a prospective, randomized comparison. *J Urol,* 157, 98-101.

Tolstunov, L., Pogrel, M. A. & Mcaninch, J. W. (1997) Intraoral morbidity following free buccal mucosal graft harvesting for urethroplasty. *Oral Surg Oral Med Oral Pathol Oral Radiol Endod,* 84, 480-2.

Vander Eeckt, K., Gontero, P. & Joniau, S. (2010) End-to-end repair or buccal mucosa graft for single-stage bulbar urethroplasty? *J Urol,* 183, e26.

Vander Eeckt, K. & Joniau, S. (2010a) End-to-end repair or buccal mucosa graft or one stage bulbar urethroplasty? *Eur Urol,* 9, 144.

Vander Eeckt, K. & Joniau, S. (2010b) Erectile function after end-to-end repair, buccal mucosa roof strip augmented anastomosis or dorsal-inlay buccal mucosa graft urethroplasty for single-stage bulbar urethroplasty *Urology.*

Vander Eeckt, K. & Joniau, S. (2010c) Postoperative morbidity of closure versus non-closure of the buccal mucosa harvest site *J Urol,* 183, E27.

Walker, D. M. (2004) Oral mucosal immunology: an overview. *Ann Acad Med Singapore,* 33, 27-30.

Wessells, H. & Mcaninch, J. W. (1996) Use of free grafts in urethral stricture reconstruction. *J Urol,* 155, 1912-5.

Wood, D. N., Allen, S. E., Andrich, D. E., Greenwell, T. J. & Mundy, A. R. (2004) The morbidity of buccal mucosal graft harvest for urethroplasty and the effect of nonclosure of the graft harvest site on postoperative pain. *J Urol,* 172, 580-3.

Wright, J. L., Wessells, H., Nathens, A. B. & Hollingworth, W. (2006) What is the most cost-effective treatment for 1 to 2-cm bulbar urethral strictures: societal approach using decision analysis. *Urology,* 67, 889-93.

Xie, H., Xu, Y. M., Xu, X. L., Sa, Y. L., Wu, D. L. & Zhang, X. C. (2009) Evaluation of erectile function after urethral reconstruction: a prospective study. *Asian J Androl,* 11, 209-14.

Yang, C. C. & Bradley, W. E. (1999) Somatic innervation of the human bulbocavernosus muscle. *Clin Neurophysiol,* 110, 412-8.

Yucel, S. & Baskin, L. S. (2003) Neuroanatomy of the male urethra and perineum. *BJU Int,* 92, 624-30.